ATLAS OF COMPUTERIZED
EMISSION TOMOGRAPHY

DEDICATED TO SIR JULES THORN

ATLAS OF COMPUTERIZED EMISSION TOMOGRAPHY

PETER JOSEF ELL MD MSc
SENIOR LECTURER, UNIVERSITY OF LONDON
CONSULTANT PHYSICIAN, MIDDLESEX HOSPITAL

JUDITH MARY DEACON MB BS MSc MRCP
REGISTRAR IN RADIOTHERAPY, ROYAL MARSDEN HOSPITAL

PETER HEDLEY JARRITT PhD
LECTURER, UNIVERSITY OF LONDON, MIDDLESEX HOSPITAL MEDICAL SCHOOL

CHURCHILL LIVINGSTONE
EDINBURGH LONDON AND NEW YORK 1980

CHURCHILL LIVINGSTONE
Medical Division of the Longman Group Limited

Distributed in the United States of America by
Churchill Livingstone Inc., 19 West 44th Street, New
York, N.Y. 10036, and by associated companies,
branches and representatives throughout the world.

First published 1980

ISBN 0 443 02228 3

British Library Cataloguing in Publication Data
Ell, Peter Josef
    Atlas of computerized emission
    tomography.
    1. Tomography – Data processing –
    I. Title   II. Deacon, Judith Mary
    III. Jarritt, Peter Hedley
    616.07′572′02854   RC78.7.T6

Printed in Great Britain by William Clowes (Beccles) Limited, Beccles and London.

PREFACE

This book describes and illustrates in detail the authors' experience in the application of single photon emission tomography. This experience was gained in an academic department of nuclear medicine attached to a major teaching hospital.

Although the instruments used are of unique design, we hope that the information provided will be of value to anyone interested in this relatively new imaging technique. An attempt has been made to describe the problems encountered in the use of emission tomography, and the relative merits of single photon or positron techniques are discussed.

Tomographic equipment is described in detail and its clinical value is analysed. Descriptions are also given of test phantoms and procedures for quality control which can be applied to comparative work with different detector configurations. We have presented 80 clinical cases, and have grouped these to illustrate the scope of single photon tomography imaging in the brain, the skull, the heart, the lungs and the liver.

An extensive bibliography is included at the end of the book.

P.J.E.
J.M.D.
P.H.J.

London, 1980

ACKNOWLEDGEMENTS

We are indebted to The Special Trustees, Middlesex Hospital and to Union Carbide for their generous grant: without it, this work would have not been possible. We are grateful to all members of our staff and in particular to our radiographers, who, throughout the years, work beyond normal routine to maintain the research spirit which permeates our nuclear medicine group; to Mary Chambers, whose secretarial help is invaluable; to all colleagues who refer patients for investigation and in particular to Dr Whiteside; and to Sir Douglas Ranger and Professor E. S. Williams for continuous support.

CONTENTS

1. INTRODUCTION: EMISSION TOMOGRAPHY

Tomographic imaging has gained widespread clinical application. The most important development in this field has been the arrival of computerized X-ray transmission tomography in 1969 (Hounsfield et al 1973). Prior to this development, however, cross-sectional image reconstruction utilizing gamma-rays instead of X-rays was successfully carried out and applied to the brain from 1963 onwards (Kuhl & Edwards 1963, Kuhl & Edwards 1968). Since then, the concept of computerized emission tomography has become increasingly familiar as a medical imaging method. The term highlights basic properties of the technique: the utilization of a computer and algorithms for image reconstruction, the emission of radiation from the organs to be imaged and the recording of tomograms, representing the distribution of the administered radiopharmaceutical within the slice (Fig. 1.1). In the last five years, a number of instruments have been developed. All have the ability to record an emission tomographic scan. Based on the type of radiation recorded (either from positron or single photon emitting radionuclides) and the number and type of radiation detectors used for the recording of the emitted radiation from the patient, they can be grouped as is shown in Table 1.1.

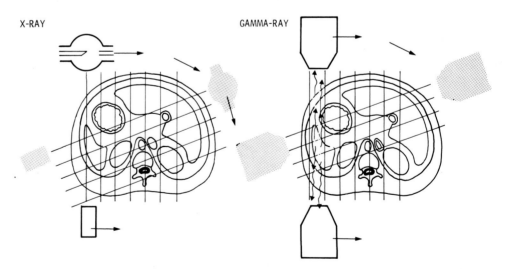

Fig. 1.1 In computerized X-ray transmission tomography, a beam of X-rays is transmitted through the body and recorded by external detectors outside it. A computer is used to calculate the difference in absorption which the X-rays undergo during their path in the body. In computerized emission tomography, once the appropriate radiopharmaceutical has been administered to the patient, gamma radiation is emitted from the body and external detectors record this information. A computer is used to reconstruct an image. This will have to take into account the attenuation of gamma-rays during their path across the body.

Table 1.1 Emission tomography imaging devices

Single Photon Single Section Detectors
Single Photon Area Detectors
Positron Single Section Detectors
Positron Area Detectors

Typically (diagrammatically shown in Fig. 1.2), emission tomographic imagers can be made of two single radiation detectors which scan the patient with rotation of the scanning assembly (one English device is an example—J & P Tomogscanner), a rotating gamma camera assembly (an Italian and American device is an example—SELO + GE) and an array of 12 or 10 radiation detectors which scan the patient at different angles without rotation of the scanning assembly (an American device is an example—Cleon-710 and 711 imagers). Special designs allow for emission tomographic imaging with positron emitting radionuclides (Phelps et al 1978, Keyes et al 1977, Ter Pogossian 1977, Muehllenher et al 1976, Brownell & Burnham 1973). Whatever instrument is used, some important advantages are obtained with this technique: recording of cross-section images with the removal of superimposed information from the adjacent structures; improvement of image contrast; utilization of radiopharmaceuticals with a quantitative assessment of their uptake, reflecting tissue metabolism and function; localization within a three-dimensional image.

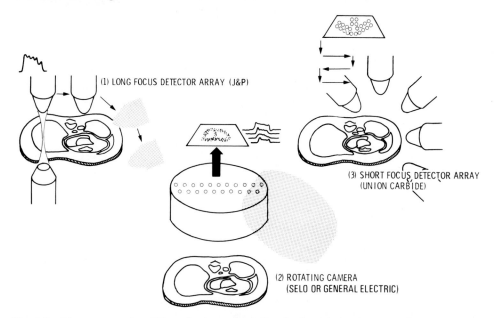

Fig. 1.2 Shows examples of three basic methods for single emission tomography instrumentation.

Removal of superimposed information

On a standard gamma camera scan, depth information from different planes of a particular organ is superimposed upon the same image. Information of interest (signal) is therefore distorted with information of less interest (noise). Theoretically, the tomographic image reconstruction allows the removal of this noise information from the tomogram cross-sectioning the region of interest (Fig. 1.3).

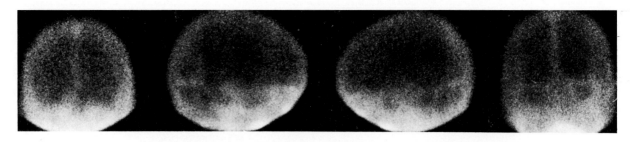

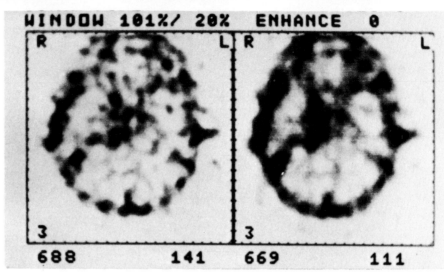

Fig. 1.3 Top row shows a 4-view study on a High Resolution Mobile Gamma Camera. No abnormality was detected.

Bottom row shows relevant tomograms. Clear outline of a large cerebello-pontine angle tumour.

Improvement of image contrast

The improvement in image contrast is a direct consequence of the improvement in the signal/noise ratio. It facilitates image interpretation but it does not necessarily improve image detail (resolution) (Fig. 1.4).

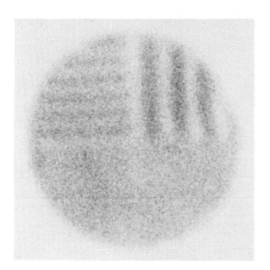

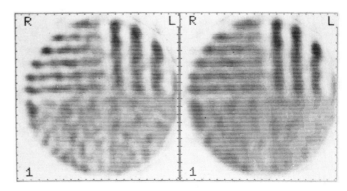

Fig. 1.4 Bar phantom imaged with conventional gamma camera (on the left) and tomographic scanner (on the right). No significant improvement in resolution is seen.

Quantification of information

This is the feature of emission tomography which may have the biggest potential in the future. An ideal system will be able to quantify accurately the amount of tracer taken up by a target organ in a unit of time. Examples of this approach are already available: the measurement of [18]Fluorine-deoxy-glucose in brain tissue (Reichvick et al 1977) and the measurement of [99m]Technetium-imidodiphosphonate uptake rates in bone (Ell et al 1978). The same principle is now also applied to the measurement of cerebral blood flow in grey or white matter with [15]Oxygen labelled blood (Subramanyan et al 1977). Quantification of information may help in the objective assessment of therapy and/or of medication over a shorter period of time.

PRESENT PROBLEMS

The arrival of a new imaging technique not only offers to the scientific and medical community potential and scope for the recording of new diagnostic information, but also tends to create a number of new problems. Some of these become progressively apparent when the new technology is making its first impact on clinical practice. The following aspects will be briefly discussed: special purpose versus general purpose instrument design, positron imaging versus single photon imaging, accuracy of image reconstruction and problems in image quantification, clinical scope and costs.

Special purpose versus general purpose design

In general, an apparatus specially designed to perform a particular task has higher chances of doing the job with success. However, considerations of cost-effectiveness have lent weight to attempts to design emission tomographic imagers based on standard equipment (scanners or gamma cameras). Trends are difficult to analyse at this stage and successful solutions (in terms of available equipment) have emerged in both directions. The positron area detectors, mainly developed in the United States, are representatives of the most sophisticated and possibly also the most expensive technology available. Resolution of 1 cm, sensitivity of data collection in the order of 50k counts/sec/μCi/cc can be achieved in special purpose designed positron imagers for the brain or small animals (Ter Pogossian et al 1978). In this case, section scanning may take as little as one second. Dynamic imaging of rapid function and/or metabolism is therefore likely to be possible in the future. Gating of data acquisition from physiological signals such as the electrocardiogram has been successfully carried out (Phelps et al 1978), with tomograms of the heart being recorded and to a large extent freed from motion artifacts. At the other end of the spectrum of emission tomographic imagers, relatively cheap and simple instruments have been developed in the U.K. The technical drawbacks will relate to very slow scanning times (of the order of 10 to 20 minutes per slice), inferior resolution (of the order of 18 mm) and low sensitivity (of the order of 5–10k counts/sec/μCi/cc). On the other hand, these devices offer an economical approach to sub-standard nuclear medicine imaging, brain and body imaging, as well as to emission tomography imaging. In terms of space occupying lesion detection and despite some interesting reports (Feine et al 1977), no data as yet is available which unequivocally shows the advantages of these latter instruments over modern gamma cameras.

Rotating gamma cameras capable of standard nuclear medicine and tomographic imaging and multidetector imagers (Jarritt et al 1979) are entering the market and penetrating imaging units away from large university centres. So far, they represent the best compromise between conflicting parameters, such as cost, versatility, patient throughput, resolution, sensitivity and ability to quantify.

Positron imaging versus single photon imaging

Positron emitters of carbon ([11]Carbon: 20 minute half-life), oxygen ([15]Oxygen: 2 minute half-life) and nitrogen ([13]Nitrogen: 10 minute half-life) are available from cyclotrons for labelling purposes. The few centres which benefit from cyclotrons programmed for the production of these radionuclides have therefore almost unlimited potential in the design and preparation of physiological tracers for imaging purposes.

Positrons are electrons having a positive electric charge which, on coming to rest, combine with an ordinary (negative) electron, the combined mass of the two particles being converted to gamma radiation. Two gamma ray photons each of 0.511 MeV are emitted in opposite directions and because of this high energy they undergo less scatter than the softer 0.140 MeV photons of [99m]Technetium. Positron detectors are therefore able to record and detect this type of radiation with greater precision and accuracy (in particular, depth independence is improved). The advantages of the use of positrons for emission tomography can be summarized:

—Improved detection with depth
—Increased statistical reliability of tomograms (due to shorter physical half-life and increased dose administration)
—More accurate quantification of information within tomograms
—Enlarged range of labelled substrates available for imaging
—Imaging of tissue specific metabolic substrates.

In Table 1.2, some examples of substrates available for positron imaging are given.

Table 1.2 Examples of substrates available for positron imaging

[18]F-Fluorodopa for studies of turnover of dopamine in brain tissue
[18]F-Fluorodeoxyglucose for studies of brain glucose metabolism
[11]C-Norepinephrine for studies of heart and fatty acid metabolism
[13]N-Ammonia for tissue perfusion studies
[77]Kr for measurements of cerebral blood flow
[11]C-Palmitic acid for studies of heart metabolism
^{68}Ga-EDTA for blood brain barrier investigations
C[15]O for blood volume studies
[15]O_2 for oxygen metabolism
[11]C-Valine for pancreatic imaging

The 'cyclotron dependence' for the production of positron emitters is clearly an important restriction to their widespread use. A longer lived positron emitter, such as [18]Fluorine, with a half-life of two hours, represents the exception, and has allowed work to be done in medical institutions not within the immediate vicinity of a cyclotron. Work with [18]Fluorine has been extensive (Subramanian et al 1975) and includes, amongst other interesting tracers, fluorosteroids to mimic hormone function, fluoropurines and fluoropyrimidines to mimic nucleic acid synthesis, fluoroamino-acids for pancreatic imaging, fluoroglucose to mimic brain metabolism. Work is in progress to further reduce this 'cyclotron dependence' on the availability of positron emitters. Generator based systems where a longer half-life parent will by elution give birth to the short-lived daughter positron-emitting nuclide are now available. Examples of such generators include:

The ^{82}Strontium–^{82}Rubidium generator: the parent isotope with a 25 day half-life, the daughter product with a 1.25 minute half-life.

The ^{68}Germanium–^{68}Gallium generator: the parent isotope with a 280 day half-life, the daughter product with a 68 minute half-life.

The main attraction in the use of single photon gamma emitters is their widespread availability. The ^{99}Molybdenum–^{99m}Technetium generator system (the parent isotope with a half-life of 68 hours, the daughter isotope with a half-life of six hours) is used worldwide in thousands of nuclear medicine centres. A whole range of radiopharmaceuticals have been introduced into clinical practice based on ^{99m}Technetium labels, forming the backbone of nuclear medicine imaging investigations. The progressive availability of ^{123}Iodine (including in the U.K., where the U.K.A.E.A. at Harwell is offering a regular supply of this material) will allow the labelling of the many substrates which lend themselves to standard iodination procedures. A new generator system—the ^{178}Tungsten–^{178}Tantalum (the parent isotope with a half-life of 22 days and the daughter isotope with a half-life of nine minutes) is now available and will further increase the range of single photon gamma imagers available for emission tomography studies. This particular isotope has the additional attraction of a very short half-life, hence allowing the use of large amounts of radioactivity (with improvement in the statistical information content of images recorded).★ Table 1.3 shows some examples of non-positron emitting radiopharmaceuticals which have been utilized in emission tomographic studies.

Table 1.3 Examples of non-positron emitting radiopharmaceuticals available for emission tomography imaging

---

^{201}Thallium for myocardial perfusion imaging
^{123}I-Hexadecanoic acid for metabolic imaging of the heart
^{123}I-Antipyrine for perfusion imaging of the brain
^{123}I-sodium iodide for research into iodine distribution
^{99m}Technetium-phosphate for the investigation of bone turnover
^{99m}Technetium-pertechnetate for the detection of space occupying disease in the brain
^{99m}Tc sulphur colloid for the detection of space occupying disease in the liver
^{99m}Tc-DMSA for the detection of space occupying disease in the kidney
^{75}Se-Cholesterol for the investigation of adrenal function
^{75}Se-Selenomethionine for the investigation of parathyroid function

---

The basic advantages of non-positron emitting radionuclides available for emission tomography include:

—The ability to be utilized with standard nuclear medicine instrumentation (scanners and gamma cameras)
—Widespread availability
—Economy
—Ease of handling in radiochemical labelling

The previous discussion and a comparison between Tables 1.2 and 1.3 betrays to some extent that non-positron emitting radiopharmaceuticals are, with few

★The most widely used short-lived isotope generator produces a single photon emitter: ^{81}Rubidium–^{81m}Krypton (parent isotope with a half-life of 4.7 hours and the daughter isotope with a half-life of 13 seconds).

exceptions, less able to mimic specific metabolic functions. Here lies their major disadvantage, although new forms of radiopharmaceutical design (liposomes, antibodies, enzyme competitors) may eventually overcome this basic restriction. In the future, much will depend on the development of new radiopharmaceuticals. If emission computerized tomography is to have an impact in clinical practice, it will have to free itself from the sophisticated university institutions and reach the regional and district hospitals. In the next five years, it is predictable that positron emission tomography is not going to achieve this. Therefore, progress or stagnation in the development of new positron emitting radionuclides and radiopharmaceuticals will dictate to a considerable extent the future scope of this new technique. It is hoped that ^{123}Iodine and the isotopes of ^{74}Bromine to ^{77}Bromine may have considerable potential in either line of development—single photon emission and positron emission.

Accuracy of image reconstruction and problems in image quantification

The ability to measure activity per unit volume is a fundamental attribute of radionuclide imaging techniques. The removal of overlying structures using transverse or longitudinal section image reconstruction has enabled this goal to be realized. However, the accuracy of such a reconstruction is dependent on many factors. Research is being carried out in order to understand the influence of the following:

    (a) Maintenance of spatial resolution across the recorded tomogram
    (b) Thickness and shape of the recorded tomogram
    (c) Uniformity of response of the radiation detectors
    (d) Attenuation of measured photons within the object
    (e) Sensitivity of the radiation detector system
    (f) Type of reconstruction algorithm used

Irrespective of the type of detection used for emission tomography (based either on single photon or positron counting), the instrument must be mechanically aligned and stable, with accurate alignment of the centre of rotation. This is of primary importance in any reconstruction technique. Errors of a few millimetres in this parameter will lead to gross artifacts. When large gamma cameras are used, the correction for non-uniform response towards an extended source of radioactivity must be undertaken and the stability of the detector system must determine how frequently this uniformity correction must be implemented. Errors of not more than 3–5 per cent must be achieved in uniformity correction.★ It is easier to achieve this aim with multiple crystals acting as detectors than it is with gamma-cameras; nevertheless, uniformity correction remains an important issue. It is vital to understand and select the appropriate reconstruction method with known resolution and noise characteristics. The input to such an algorithm must necessarily possess a satisfactory signal to noise ratio (with insufficient data, reconstruction will be suboptimal or will lead to excessive data collection time); therefore, relative sensitivities of each detector system will determine the length of time required for data collection. Little data is available with regard to the errors expected in a reconstructed image and is limited to iterative and/or convolution techniques. For images containing one million detected events, the expected root mean square uncertainty may be as high as 25 per cent, although this figure will be

★(If 'ring' artifacts are not to appear in the tomographic imager).

modified by any attenuation conditions which have to be applied. Attenuation corrections are usually based on transmission data. However, this is mostly applicable to a non-focussing detector system. The implications of these errors on accurate quantification for radioactive distributions is obvious. Nevertheless, the physical data available relates only to extended objects, i.e., objects within which the activity distribution is uniform for thicknesses at least twice that of the detected slice. Further errors can be introduced when corrections have to be made for a non-uniform slice thickness and a varying spatial resolution within the slice which will limit the area over which quantification of activity can be contemplated. Even when all these factors have been taken into account and have been mathematically solved, the clinical situation is different. Here, one is often faced with activity distributions which are not equivalent to phantom conditions. In tomograms adjacent to the slice being imaged, areas of high activity may exist and will contribute to the activities measured within the slice of interest; this contribution is at this stage still difficult to quantify but it may be large.

Table 1.4 Spatial resolution

	FWHM	Typical scanning times in minutes
Positron tomography (Ortec ECAT)	14–17 mm	1–4 per slice
Rotating GE camera	15–20 mm	10–20 (all slices)
Rotating 2 head Searle	16 mm	10–20 (all slices)
Cleon-710 head scanner	9 mm	4 per slice
Cleon-711 body scanner	21–23 mm	5 per slice
J & P Tomogscanner	17–20 mm	10–15 per slice

Table 1.4 offers approximate values for Full Width Half Maximum (FWHM) for a number of instruments.

CLINICAL SCOPE

Clinical work on emission computerized tomography is seeking new data in two major areas: in the field of space occupying lesion detection and in the field of functional and metabolic studies.

Space occupying lesion detection

If emission tomographic imaging is going to succeed in this field, it will have to take into account present levels of accuracy, sensitivity and specificity of the existing and well-established imaging techniques: standard radiology, nuclear medicine, ultrasound and computerized X-ray tomography. It will have to prove itself as a method of superior detection capability or as a method which records valuable information from organs which so far escape ideal imaging with existing technology. This task is clearly a difficult one. Considerations such as imaging time and overall cost will have to be accounted for. Ideally, emission tomography should replace rather than be added to a standard nuclear medicine imaging protocol for space occupying lesion detection. So far, no clear picture has emerged but some trends can be analysed.

The brain. Despite the obvious success of X-ray transmission tomography, nuclear medicine brain scans are performed in hundreds (in the U.K.) and thousands of centres worldwide. The reasons for this can be found in the economy, speed, low radiation exposure and high accuracy of detection of malignant disease, established cerebrovascular disease, and chronic subdural haematomata. Nuclear medicine brain scanning is an important clinical tool and it will remain so for many years to come. Can emission tomography help?

In our experience, emission tomographic imaging of the brain increases the accuracy, sensitivity and specificity of space occupying lesion detection compared with standard nuclear medicine investigations. It can, with success, replace standard gamma camera imaging, in particular in the detection of primary neoplasms, single or multiple secondaries and chronic subdural haematomata. We have experience in more than 200 patients that a combination of a one minute dynamic perfusion study of the brain at the time of intravenous administration of the tracer followed by a 30 minute emission tomography imaging procedure can be a substitute for traditional gamma camera imaging. In this case, emission tomography does not add to overall imaging time in the investigation of patients. In some instances, and in particular cerebrovascular disease, additional gamma camera views are still required, but time is saved with this new approach in a busy nuclear medicine referral centre.

The clinical case material offered in this atlas shows that emission computerized tomography (CET) can detect more lesions than those found with conventional 2-D gamma-camera imaging and that localization of lesions is significantly improved with this new approach.

Work has been carried out concerning imaging of the ventricle spaces and studies of CSF flow. The value of emission tomography has been demonstrated in the evaluation of cerebrospinal fluid (CSF) pathways, definition of pools of abnormal CSF, hydrocephalus, cistern deformities, etc. Sequential scanning with time has proven to be of particular value in differentiating CSF stasis from normal flows (Rothenberg et al, 1976, Wooley et al 1977).

The liver. The detection of space occupying lesions of the liver is performed routinely via nuclear medicine, ultrasound and computerized X-ray tomography. None of these techniques is 100 per cent accurate, sensitive and specific. The techniques appear to have similar advantages and disadvantages (Alfidi et al 1976, Bayan et al 1977, Bragg 1977, Cosgrove & McCready 1978), such that the outcome of comparative studies leads to a familiar conclusion in medicine: 'These tests are complementary rather than competitive.' Nevertheless, taking factors such as imaging time, cost, radiation dosimetry, predictive values, and others into account, a strategy for the detection of space occupying disease in the liver is emerging (Ell et al 1978). Can emission tomography help?

A firm answer cannot be given at this stage. Although clinical data is already available pointing at an increase of lesion detectability (Carril et al 1978, Firusian 1978), questions remain in abeyance for further research. Nuclear medicine liver imaging is, in contrast with brain imaging, a method of 'cold spot' detection. The available radiopharmaceuticals concentrate in areas of normal tissue and enable the detection of pathology by their absence in pathological tissue. The problems are similar to those encountered in liver contrast angiography, where more often than desirable, lesions are only detected by noting the displacement of vessels rather than by the imaging of a perfusion blush (the vascularity of lesions in the liver is known to be poor). The irregularity of size and shape of livers represents an additional difficulty when considering an emission tomography approach. Sections of this organ which will not cover the entire dimensions of the liver may lead to difficulties in interpretation and a rise in the false positive rate (the problem to overcome in nuclear medicine liver scanning). Whether emission tomography of the liver will replace standard techniques of scanning of this organ remains to be seen.

The kidney. Most lesions of the kidney are conventionally detected on routine IVP and/or ultrasound scanning. Only a small percentage of patients will require further diagnostic work-up (in terms of lesion detection) and these will proceed to transmission X-ray tomography and/or angiography. Nevertheless, a small percentage of patients remain difficult to diagnose. Not always can an IVP be performed and in approximately 10 per cent of cases ultrasound imaging provides insufficient data. Renal scanning with radiopharmaceuticals has been significantly improved with the appearance of tracers such as [99m]Technetium-DMSA (dimercaptosuccinic acid) and images with high information density can be recorded. Since the contour and shape of the kidneys is fairly regular, emission tomography is made easier. Even with 'cold spot' detection (as it happens for the kidney) emission tomograms of reasonable detail can be recorded (Fig. 1.5). However, the clinical implications of this approach remain unexplored and data will have to be collected in order to ascertain the viability of the technique.

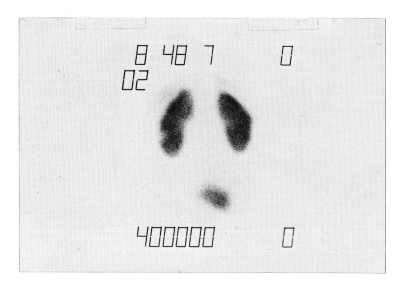

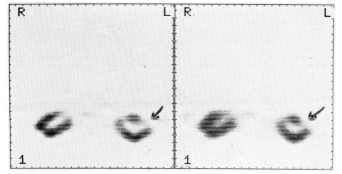

Fig. 1.5 Top row shows gamma camera image. Kidneys of piglet imaged with a 9 mm lesion implanted in left renal cortex.
Bottom row shows tomographic image. Note clear outline of lesion.

Other organs. The thyroid, parathyroids, pancreas, adrenals and prostate, lungs, heart, mediastinum, lymph nodes and retroperitoneal space represent organs and spaces where space occupying disease can occur. The impact of emission tomographic imaging is in these areas in its infancy. Clinical trials might show that in certain circumstances the new approach will bear fruit. In a situation of high background with relatively poor uptake of the radiopharmaceutical in the organ or area of interest, emission tomography may well result in better localization and definition of the organ to be imaged. This could lead to improved staging of tumours with agents such as ^{67}Gallium-citrate, improved localization of adenomata with ^{75}Selenium-selenomethionine, and so on.

Functional and metabolic studies

In this area, emission tomography is expected to make significant contributions in the understanding of a variety of organ functions and patterns of metabolism. The discussion concerning the utilization of positrons has already pointed at the potential of this new technique. From all the generator systems mentioned and available to produce positron emitters, the ^{68}Germanium–^{68}Gallium appears to be the most interesting one. This is not to say that this generator has achieved maturity; although already commercially available, it offers ^{68}Gallium in a chelate form. Systems attempting to produce ^{68}Gallium in an ionic form still require development and refinement. So far, clinically interesting pharmaceuticals based on ^{68}Gallium are still awaiting development. Brain, liver and lung studies have been performed but not to advantage when compared with standard procedures.

Positron emitters such as ^{11}C, ^{15}O, ^{13}N and ^{18}F are the source of a wealth of interesting data. Brain, heart and pulmonary function are under investigation with these radionuclides. The measurement of glucose consumption of the brain and the heart, the estimation of oxygen transport to different body tissues, the analysis of tissue perfusion, rate and change with time or treatment, the investigation of liver pathology with ^{13}N-labelled ammonia and ^{13}N-labelled alanine for pancreatic imaging, measurements of extravascular lung water, splenic red blood cell mass, fatty acid turnover in the heart, studies involving ^{11}Carbon-labelled psychotropic drugs (chlorpromazine, imipramine, diazepam) give an indication of the variety, interest and potential of the new methodology. ^{18}Fluorine-labelled compounds such as phenylalanine, tyrosine, Dopa, tryptophan, haloperidol, further show the present research and clinical potential.

Non-positron gamma emitters and tomographic imaging have also been employed in the analysis of organ function and metabolism. Examples can be given in the use of ^{201}Thallium in the detection of myocardial ischaemia, of ^{123}Iodine-labelled hexadecanoic acid in the study of cardiac fatty acid turnover, of ^{99m}Technetium-labelled phosphates in the evaluation of metabolic bone disease, of ^{123}Iodine-antipyrine in cerebral perfusion studies, of ^{81m}Krypton perfusion studies of the brain, the heart and the lungs, and so on.

Investigation of organ or tissue specific metabolism or function, objective assessment through quantification and three-dimensional imaging of tomograms of the body, summarize the inherent potential of computerized emission tomography. The measurement of uptake of a physiological tracer or analogue in terms of μCi of tracer administered per unit of tissue volume per unit of time, or the measurement of flow per g of tissue per unit of time are sufficiently exciting to motivate scientists and clinicians into further research in this field. The years to come will indeed be stimulating.

COSTS

It is important to finalize this review with a note of caution. So far, computerized emission tomography is expensive and not cost-effective. The long dreamed 'desk-top' cyclotron for medical purposes has now reached the production stage. Its cost remains, however, high and in the order of £500 000 to £700 000. A team of experts will be required to man and run the machine with increased demands on resources. Finally, positron tomographic imagers and other instrumentation designed for emission tomography remains very costly (in the order of £100 000 to £500 000). The infrastructure for the labelling of short-lived radiopharmaceuticals with large amounts of radioactivity is also a technically complex and costly exercise. It will take years before this new methodology unequivocally demonstrates its clinical usefulness. In the meantime, however, and in a few centres, research in this field must be allowed to continue.

Whether or not single photon emission tomography will establish itself as a relevant clinical tool is fundamentally linked to future work: primarily on the development of improved biological tracers and secondarily on the improvement of reconstruction algorithms which will accurately reflect the *in vivo* 3-dimensional distribution of these tracers. In relative terms and from these two aspects of the methodology, the instrumentation is ahead of its time.

There appears to be a place for special purpose designed instrumentation (e.g. brain imaging and paediatric body scanning). There is also a place for general purpose systems based on modern scintillation detectors (e.g. gamma camera) and these may turn out to be the most cost effective. From a clinical input point of view, scanning times of the order of 2–4 minutes/slice are the longest acceptable. FWHM of the order of 15 mm or less may represent a minimum requirement for the recording of clinically relevant data.

REFERENCES

Alfidi R J, Haaga J R, Havrilla T H, Pepe R G, Cook S A 1976 Computed tomography of the liver. American Journal of Radiology 127: 69

Bayan P J, Dinn W M, Grossman Z D, Wistow B W, McAfee J G, Kieffer S A 1977 Correlation of computed tomography, grey scale ultrasonography and radionuclide imaging of the liver in detecting space occupying processes. Radiology 124 (2): 387

Bragg D G 1977 Advances in diagnostic radiology: problems and prospects. Cancer 40, 1:500, 8

Brownell G L, Burnham C A 1973 In: Tomographic Imaging in Nuclear Medicine, Friedman, New York, Society of Nuclear Medicine

Carril J M, Dendy P P, MacDonald A F, Keyes W I, Undrill P E, Mallard J R 1978 Results of prospective trials for clinical evaluation of radioisotope emission tomography of the brain and liver. European Society of Nuclear Medicine, Second Congress, London.

Cosgrove D O, McCready V R 1978 Diagnosis of liver metastases using ultrasound and isotope scanning techniques. Journal of the Royal Society of Medicine 71: 652

Ell P J, Jarritt P H, Deacon J M, Brown N J G, Williams E S 1978 Emission computerized tomography—a new imaging technique. The Lancet II: 608–610

Ell P J, Williams E S, Todd-Pokropek A E 1978 The clinical use of diagnostic imaging. British Journal of Hospital Medicine 20, 2: 119–127

Feine U, Anger K, Müller-Schauenburg W, Milward R C 1977 Erste klinische Erfahrungen mit einem axialen Emissions-Computer-Tomographen. Röfo 127, 4: 358-365

Firusian N 1978 Transversal-section investigation of liver by using gamma-ray computer tomography. European Society of Nuclear Medicine. Second Congress, London

Hounsfield G, Ambrose H, Perry J, Bridges C 1973 Computerized transverse axial scanning. British Journal of Radiology 46: 1016-1051

Jarritt P H, Ell P J, Myers M, Brown N J G, Deacon J M 1979 A new transverse section brain imager. Journal of Nuclear Medicine 20: 319-327

Keyes J W, Orelandea N, Heetderks W J et al 1977 The humongotron—a scintillation camera transaxial tomograph. Journal of Nuclear Medicine 18: 381–387

Kuhl D E, Edwards R G 1963 Image separation radioisotope scanning. Radiology 80: 653–661

Kuhl D E, Edwards R G 1968 Recognizing data from transverse sections of the brain using digital processing. Radiology 91: 975–983

Muehllenhner G, Buchin N P, Dubek G H 1976 Performance parameters of the positron imaging camera. IEEE Nuclear Scientist 23: 528–537

Phelps M E, Hoffman E J, Huang S-C, Kuhl D E 1978 ECAT: A new computerized tomographic imaging system for positron-emitting radiopharmaceuticals. The Journal of Nuclear Medicine 19, 6: 635–647

Phelps M E, Hoffman E J, Huang S-C 1978 Physiologic tomography. World Federation of Nuclear Medicine and Biology, Second International Congress, Washington

Reichvick M, Kuhl D E, Wolf A 1977 Measurement of local cerebral glucose metabolism in man with ^{18}F-deoxy-D-glucose in cerebral function, metabolism and circulation. Ingvar and Lassen, Copenhagen, Munksgaard, 190–191

Rothenberg H P, Devenney J, Kuhl D E 1976 Transverse section radionuclide scanning in cisternography. Journal of Nuclear Medicine. 17, 924–929

Subramanian G, Rhodes B A, Cooper J F, Sodd U S 1975 Radiopharmaceuticals. Society of Nuclear Medicine. (ISBN 0–88416–041–6)

Subramanyan R, Bucelewicz W M, Hoop B Jr, Jones S C 1977 A system for oxygen-15 labelled blood for medical applications. The International Journal of Applied Radiation and Isotopes 28, 1/2: 21–24

Ter Pogossian M M 1977 Basic principles of computed axial tomography. Seminars in Nuclear Medicine 7: 109–127

Ter Pogossian M M, Mullani N A, Hood J T, Higgins C S, Fiche D C 1978 Design considerations for a positron emission transverse tomograph (PETTV) for imaging of the brain. Journal of Computer Assisted Tomography 2: 539–544

Wooley J L, Williams B, Venkatesh 1977 Cranial Isotopic Section Scanning. Clinical Radiology 28: 517–528

2. ATLAS OF CLINICAL APPLICATIONS

MATERIALS AND METHODS

All brain scans were performed on the Cleon-710 tomographic scanner.

Dose: 15 mCi of $^{99m}TcO_4^-$
Window Setting: 130–170 keV
Scan Time: 4 minutes/slice
Background Cut-off: 25 per cent
Slice Spacing: 1.25 cm
Frame Tilt: variable
Imaging Time: 60 min post injection

Dynamic perfusion sequence (3 sec images) and static gamma camera images on high resolution 37-photomultiplier tube Nuclear Enterprises, Searle Radiographics or Ohio Nuclear cameras.

X-ray transmission scans on EMI CT5005 scanner.

All skull, liver and spleen, chest and heart scans were performed on the Cleon-711 tomographic scanner. Standard doses and radiopharmaceuticals were used. Identical technical set-up as for Cleon-710, except:

Slice Spacing: 2.0 cm
Scan Time: 5 minutes/slice

Whole Body Bone Scans performed on the Cleon-760 whole body scanner.

Annotation used
CET: computerized emission tomography (Cleon-710 or 711)
CTT: computerized transmission tomography (EMI CT5005)
AP, PA, RL, LL = anterior, posterior, right lateral and left lateral projections.

Brain: normal anatomy and physiology

Patient 1

Clinical history

This 35-year-old woman presented with a pigmented naevus on the right thigh which had been growing larger for about a year.

Malignant melanoma was diagnosed on biopsy, and the lesion was widely excised.

A brain scan was requested as a routine screening test in the process of staging the disease.

Imaging

CET scan. Note normal tomograms, recorded from the base to the convexity of the skull.

Emission tomography allows for the definition of the anterior, middle and posterior cerebral fossae. The orbits, foramen magnum, cavernous sinuses, sigmoid, transverse and sagittal sinuses are well seen. There is dramatic improvement in the definition of these structures over that recorded with conventional Anger gamma camera imaging.

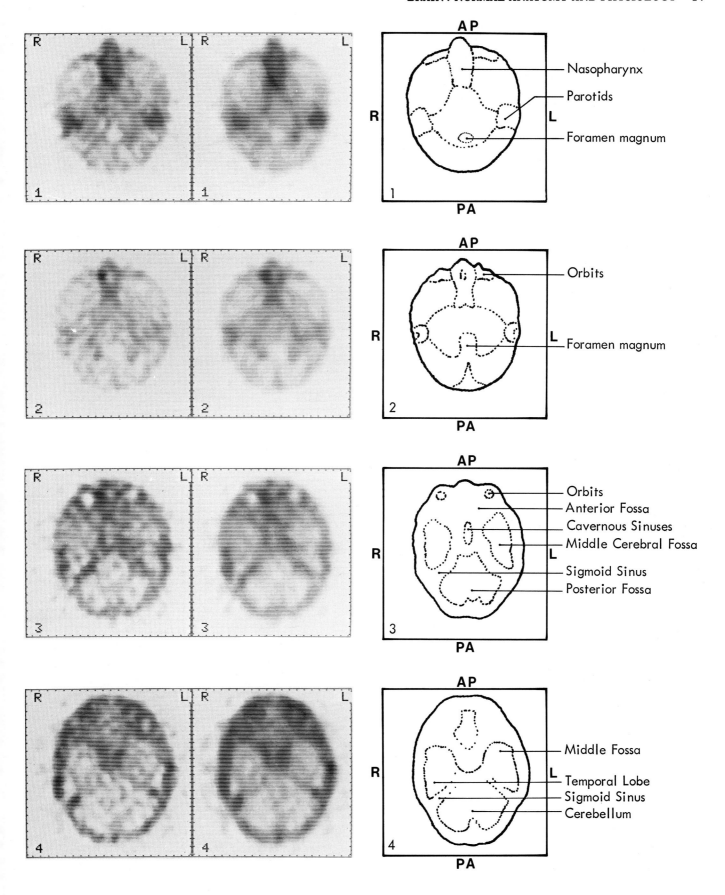

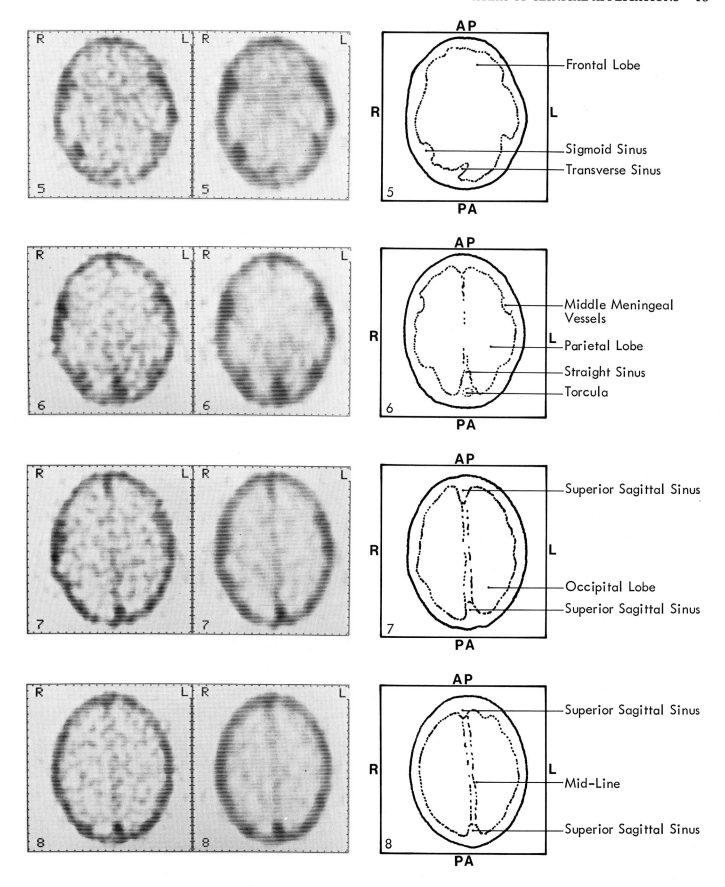

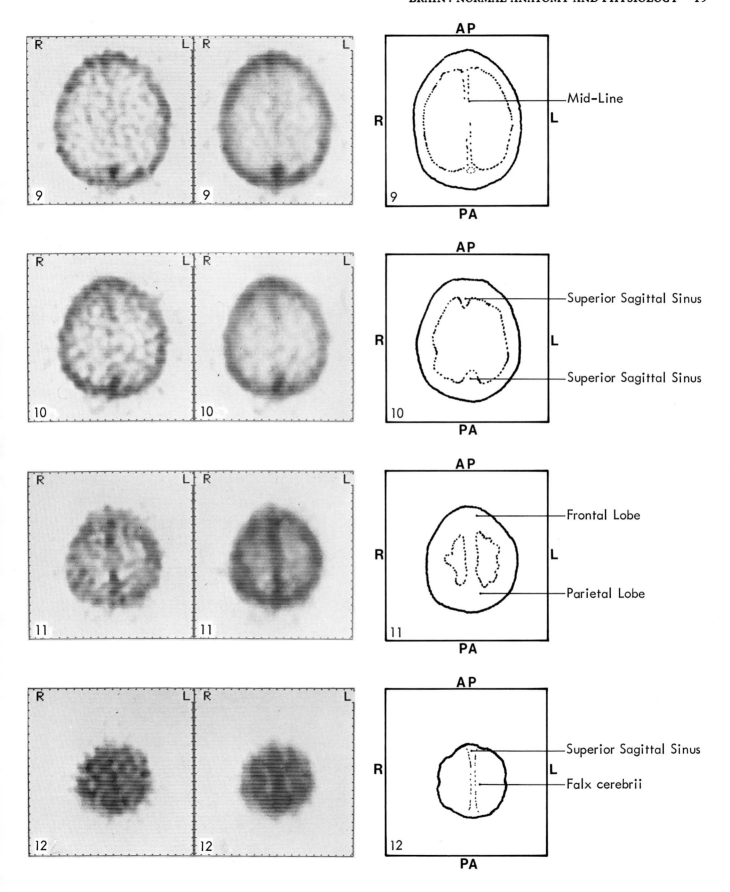

Patient 2

Clinical history

This 25-year-old woman from El Salvador had been in the United Kingdom for three years. Since the age of nine years, she had occasional grand mal epileptic fits, which had been well controlled with anticonvulsants. There was no family history of epilepsy, and no history of birth trauma.

Since immigration, she had discontinued her anticonvulsant therapy and had since suffered migrainous headaches and six grand mal fits.

Clinical examination was normal. EEG—normal.

Imaging

CET scan. Normal tomograms of the brain. Note the reproducibility in the definition of normal anatomy and physiology in the emission tomograms of these first two case examples.

Final diagnosis

Idiopathic epilepsy.

Outcome

She responded well to reinstitution of anticonvulsants.

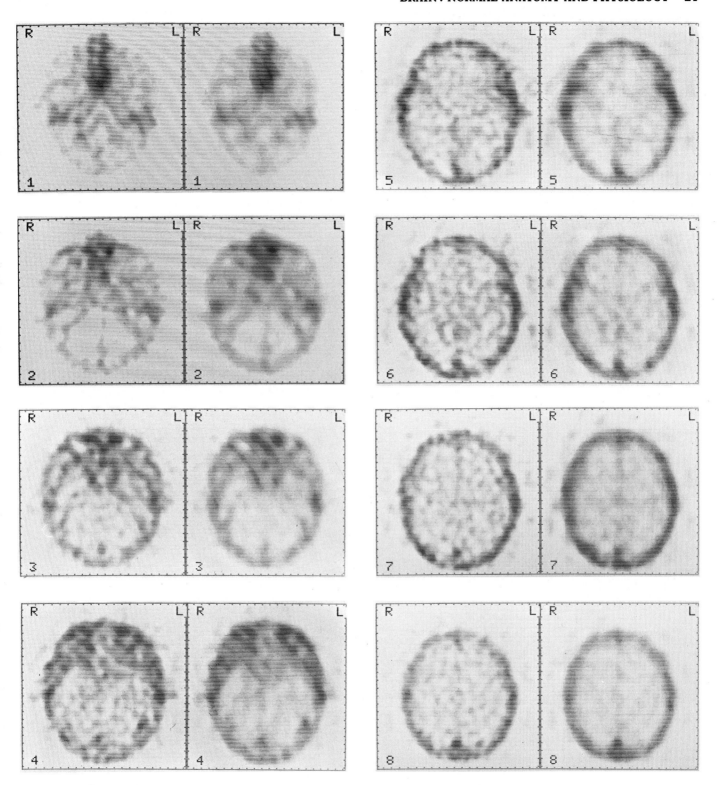

Patient 3

CET scan showing normal distribution of ^{99m}Tc red cells

Dose: 15 mCi ^{99m}Tc
Scanning Time/Slice: 4 minutes
$\frac{1}{2}$ inch slice spacing

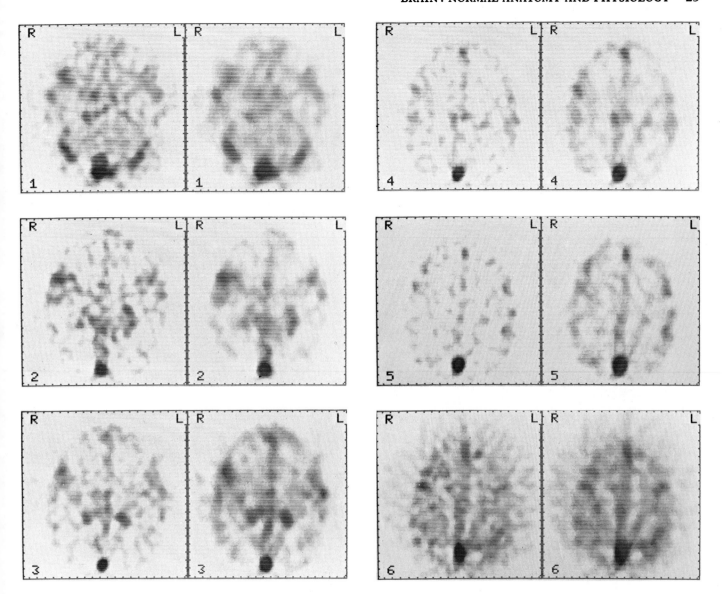

Brain: vascular disease

Patient 4

Clinical history

This 70-year-old woman had a 5 year history of carcinoma of the cervix, treated with surgery and radiotherapy, and had since been well with no signs of recurrence or metastases. She presented after an episode of transient paraesthesia in her right arm, accompanied by dysphasia. There were no abnormal neurological signs.

Provisional diagnosis. Possible cerebral metastases, or transient ischaemic attack.

Imaging

Brain scan. The dynamic gamma camera study showed peripheral flattening over the convexity of the left cerebral hemisphere.

CET scan one hour later showed a well defined crescent of increased activity over the high convexity of the left parietal region. These findings were confirmed on a static gamma camera view.

On further questioning, the patient gave a history of a fall, four weeks prior to the investigation, in which she had hit her head, but had not lost consciousness or suffered obvious sequelae.

Final diagnosis

Subdural haematoma in the left parietal convexity.

Outcome

Subdural haematoma was evacuated through burr-holes and the patient made a rapid and complete recovery.

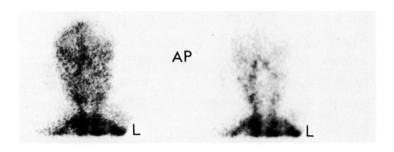

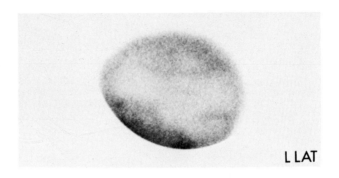

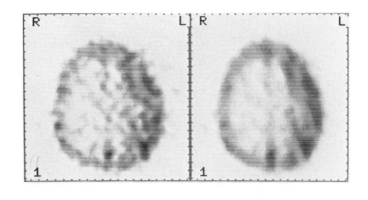

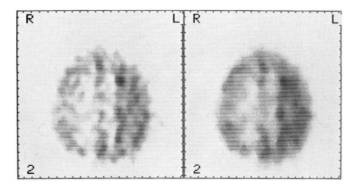

Patient 5

Clinical history

This 24-year-old girl was admitted with sudden onset of severe headache and neck stiffness. At the ages of 10 and 13 years, she had suffered episodes of subarachnoid haemorrhage, from which she had recovered spontaneously. Lumbar puncture produced heavily bloodstained CSF.

Provisional diagnosis. Recurrent subarachnoid haemorrhage.

Imaging

Brain scan. The dynamic study showed a marked blush of activity close to the mid-line. An immediate static gamma camera view confirmed a persistent area of increased activity in the right parietal region.

CET scan showed increased activity in the region of the right mid-brain, extending posteriorly to the superior saggital sinus.

CTT scan showed the same abnormality in the relevant cuts.

Carotid angiography showed a deep right parietal A–V malformation, in the region of the thalamus, fed by four large arteries, and with a large posteriorly draining vein.

Final diagnosis

Large arteriovenous malformation.

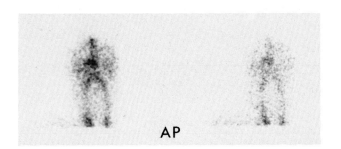

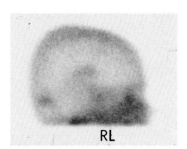

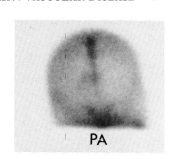

AP

RL

PA

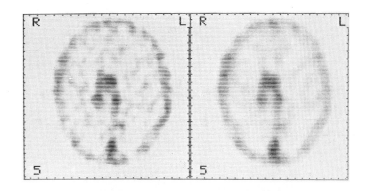

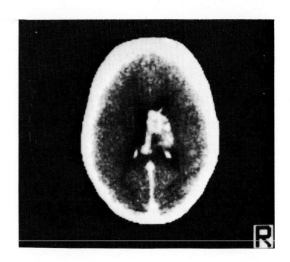

Patient 6

Clinical history	This 63-year-old man first presented with a mild right sided weakness, which slowly resolved over a period of days. Three months later, he was admitted with a dense right hemiplegia, expressive dysphasia and a right homonymous hemianopia.
	Provisional diagnosis. Left sided cerebro-vascular accident (CVA).
Imaging	*Brain scan.* Dynamic study showed severe underperfusion of the whole of the left side of the brain. Static gamma camera views showed increased activity in the territory of the anterior and posterior cerebral arteries on the left, and also in the temporal region.
	CET scan confirmed that most of the left cerebral hemisphere showed abnormal uptake of tracer. Note improved definition of the extent of involvement on the tomographic study.
Final diagnosis	Extensive left sided CVA.

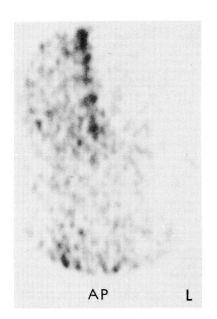

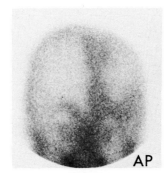

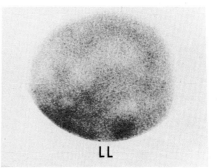

AP   L   AP   LL

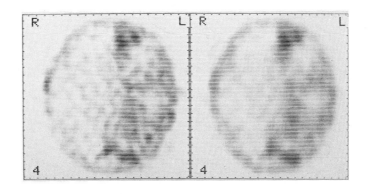

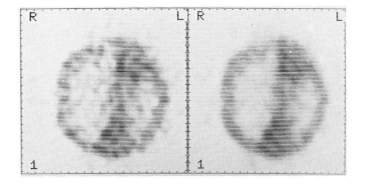

Patient 7

Clinical history

This 63-year-old man was admitted with mild congestive cardiac failure, associated with rapid atrial fibrillation.

He had a past history of syphilitic aortitis with aortic regurgitation diagnosed 17 months previously and treated with penicillin. Maturity onset diabetes was discovered at the same time and treated with diet. Eight days after admission, he developed a dense left sided weakness of sudden onset.

Provisional diagnosis. Cerebral embolism.

Imaging

CET scan showed an extensive area of increased activity occupying the majority of the right temporal and parietal lobes. The shape of the lesion and its position suggested a large CVA in the territory of the middle cerebral artery. The emission scan gives a more precise definition of the extent of the lesion in depth, its relationship with neighbouring structures and the midline.

CTT scan showed an enhancing area of reduced attenuation in the same region.

Final diagnosis

Right middle cerebral CVA, probably embolic.

Outcome

There was some improvement in movements of the left leg over the next eight weeks, but the upper limb remained flaccid.

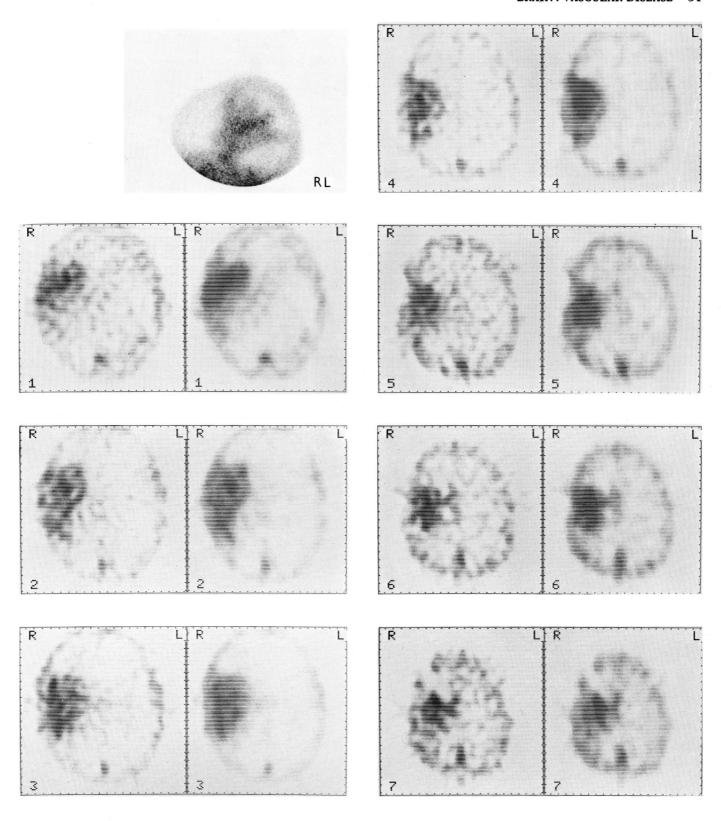

Patient 8

Clinical history	This 71-year-old man was admitted as an emergency having been found at home semiconscious. He had been well the previous evening but was known to have fallen and hit his head three days previously. He was known to be a heavy drinker, and had a history of blackouts of uncertain aetiology.
On examination	He was semiconscious, there was a complete aphasia, right homonymous hemianopia and a dense right sided hemiplegia.
	Provisional diagnosis. CVA or possible subdural haematoma.
Imaging	*Brain scan* showed abnormal activity in the left temporoparietal region.
	CET scan showed an area of increased activity in the left temporoparietal region, extending from the periphery into the substance of the hemisphere, compatible with a cerebral infarct. No evidence of a subdural haematoma.
Final diagnosis	Left middle cerebral artery CVA.
Outcome	The patient made a rapid recovery, the hemiplegia resolving within three days, but a slight dysphasia remained.

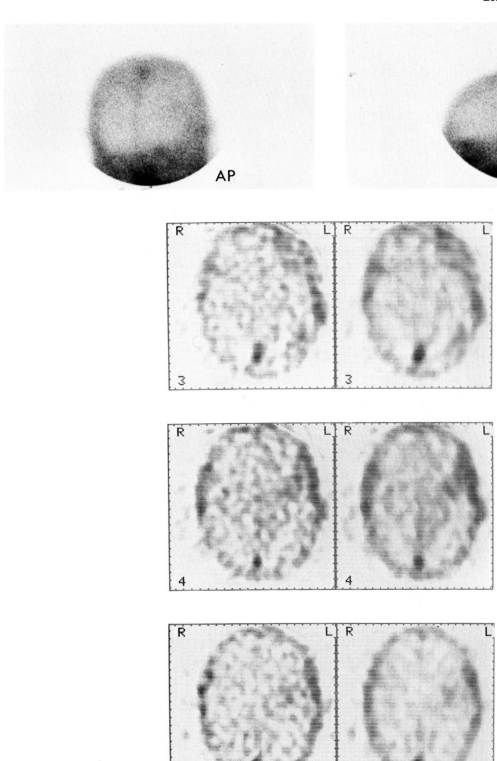

Patient 9

Clinical history This 75-year-old man was admitted with sudden onset of left sided weakness. One month previously, he had suffered an episode of loss of consciousness, followed by a transient left hemianopia, facial palsy and hemiparesis, which recovered within 24 hours.

On examination There was a left sided hemiparesis and frontal lobe signs with the presence of primitive reflexes.

Provisional diagnosis. Cerebral infarction.

Imaging *Brain scan.* There was increased activity in the right posterior parietal region.

CET scan showed extensive areas of abnormal activity extending from the right temporal lobe posteriorly into the right parieto-occipital region. This activity extended high into the occipital lobe and was classically wedge-shaped.

Final diagnosis Right parietal and occipital infarction.

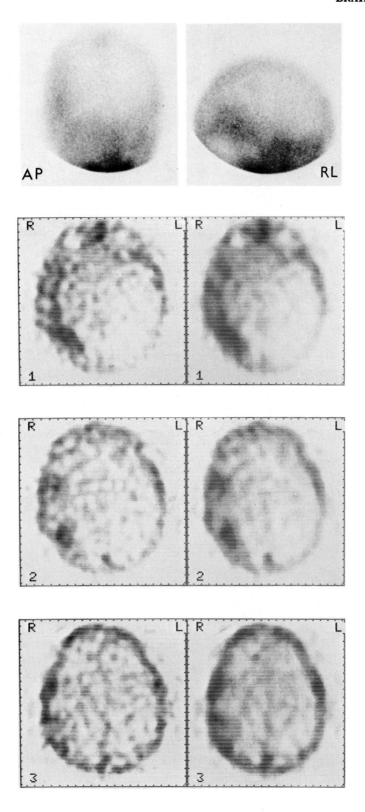

Patient 10

Clinical history   This 76-year-old man presented with sudden onset of severe left sided weakness.

On examination   There was a dense left sided hemiplegia, with a left sided facial palsy.

Provisional diagnosis. Right parietal CVA.

Imaging   *CET* scans were performed at one and at four days after the incident. On day one, there was a very slight degree of increased activity in the right parietal region. The scan on day four showed a marked, wedge-shaped area of abnormal activity in the right parietal region.

CTT scans performed on the same days showed an extensive low attenuation area in the right middle cerebral artery territory, which did not enhance, and did not change in appearance over the period of study.

Final diagnosis   Large right parietal infarct.

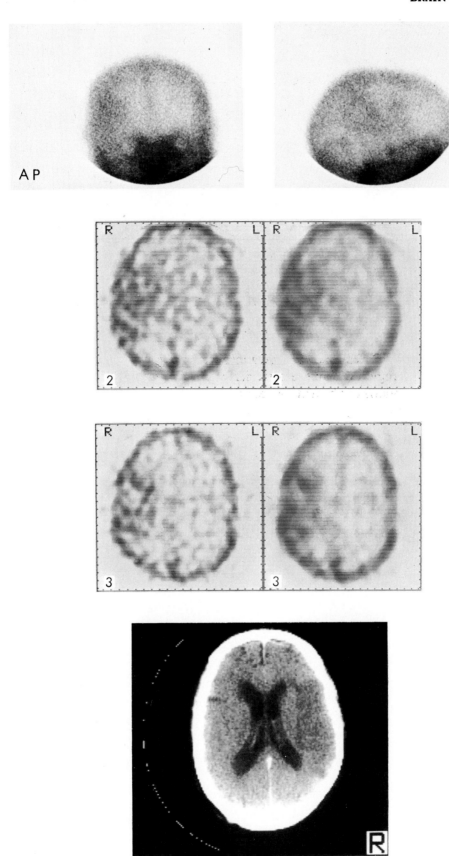

Patient 11

Clinical history   This 43-year-old woman was admitted for removal of a benign ovarian cyst. Two days post-operatively, she complained of sudden onset of unsteadiness and generalized weakness.

On examination   She was found to have a mild right sided weakness and right homonymous hemianopia.

Provisional diagnosis. Left sided CVA.

Imaging   *CET scan* showed an extensive area of increased uptake in the left occipital region within the posterior cerebral artery territory. The static gamma camera views confirmed the lesion.

CTT scan showed mixed attenuation in the left occipital region which enhanced with contrast.

Cerebral angiography showed a posterior cerebral artery CVA, probably embolic.

Final diagnosis   Posterior cerebral artery CVA.

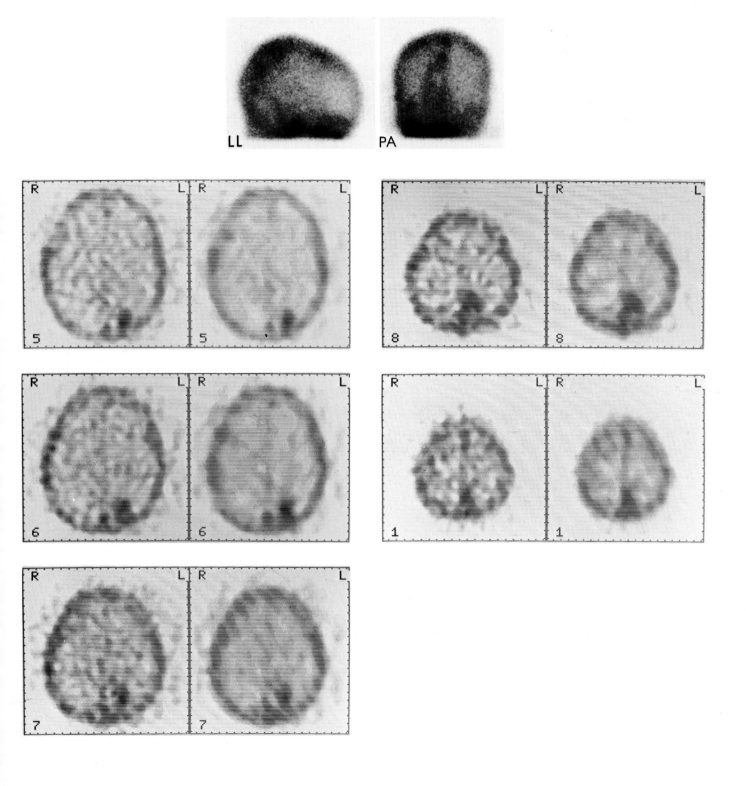

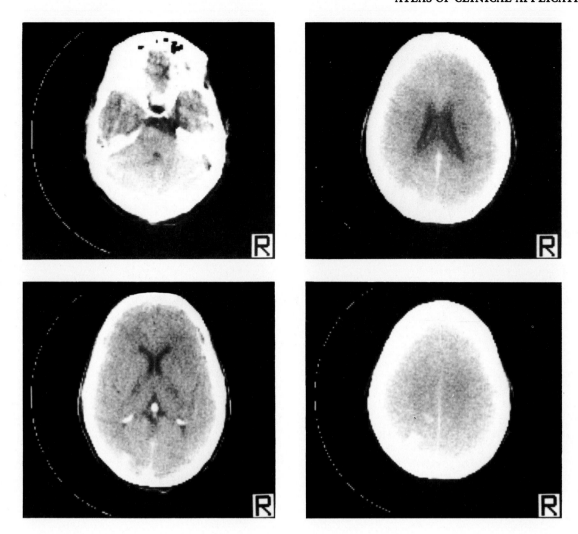

Patient 12

Clinical history	This 77-year-old woman presented with nominal dysphasia, and transient episodes of aphasia.
On examination	She was dysphasic and dysgraphic with right/left disorientation and right sided inattention. There was a mild right hemiparesis. A large left sphenoidal wing meningioma was found on carotid angiography and was removed at craniotomy. Three days post-operatively, the patient developed a dense right hemiplegia and severe dysphasia.
	Provisional diagnosis. Post-operative cerebral infarction.
Imaging	*CET scan* showed a large wedge-shaped area of abnormal activity in the left temporoparietal region compatible with a middle cerebral artery CVA.
	CTT scan showed low attenuation in the deep left middle cerebral artery distribution, compatible with an infarct.
Outcome	The patient made a very slow recovery and moderate right sided weakness and dysphasia persisted.

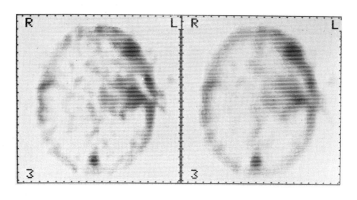

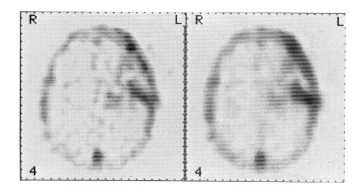

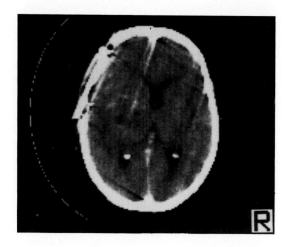

Brain: Tuberculoma

Patient 13

Clinical history

This 27-year-old girl presented with a seven month history of cough, haemoptysis, loss of weight and night sweats. There was a right sided pleural effusion and several fluctuant lumps on her back and legs. A diagnosis of tuberculosis was made on sputum culture and antituberculous chemotherapy was instituted. Ten days later, she suffered one grand mal fit, followed by a left sided Jacksonian fit. The CSF was normal. There were no abnormal neurological signs.

Provisional diagnosis. Possible cerebral tuberculoma.

Imaging

Dynamic brain scan. Normal.

CET scan. A small round area of increased activity was seen in the right temporoparietal region.

Final diagnosis

Tuberculoma.

Outcome

Phenytoin was instituted and antituberculous treatment was continued. The patient's condition steadily improved and she suffered no further fits.

A repeat CET scan two months later was normal.

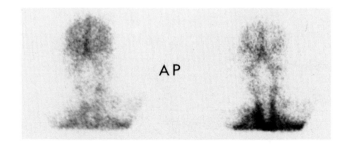

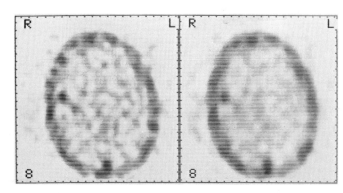

Brain: malignant disease (primary)

Patient 14

Clinical history   This 71-year-old female patient had a six week history of ataxia and vertigo, with right sided fifth, eighth and partial seventh nerve symptoms.

Imaging   *Brain scan.* Standard 4-view gamma camera scan shows an area of increased tracer uptake, round and well defined, in the vicinity of the cerebellopontine angle. The relationship of this lesion with the neighbouring brain structures is still not entirely clearcut.

CET and CTT scans. The lesion is well seen and its relationship with neighbouring structures very apparent. Note the similarity between CET and CTT scans.

Final diagnosis   Right cerebello-pontine angle tumour.

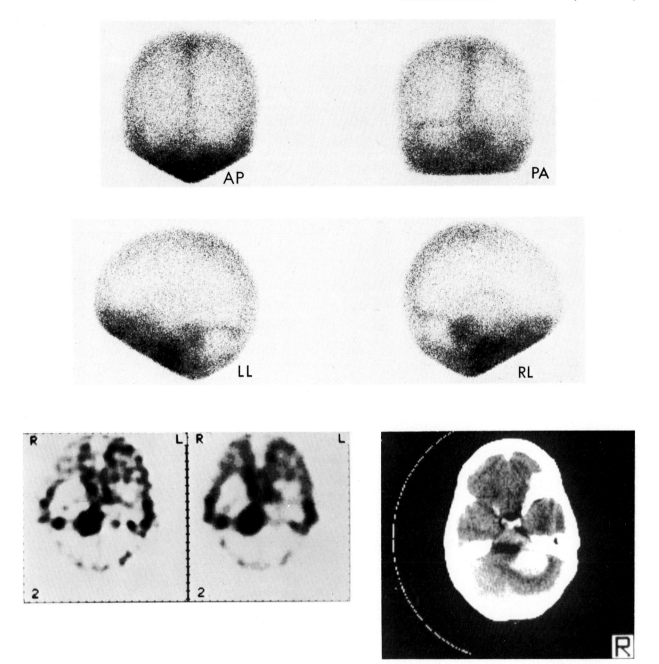

Patient 15

Clinical history

This 44-year-old male was admitted for further investigation of a possible space occupying lesion in the brain. Four months previously, he had an episode of left sided Jacksonian fits, followed by weakness of the left arm and hand. There was persistent upper motor neurone weakness of the left arm and hand, paraesthesia of the left arm and extensor plantar responses.

Imaging

CTT scans. Two scans were performed (with and without contrast) and both investigations *were normal.*

Carotid angiogram. A right carotid angiogram was performed and also considered *normal.*

CET scan. A single, large, well defined and round *lesion* was found in the *right parietal lobe.*

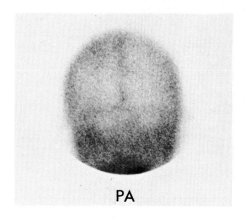

PA

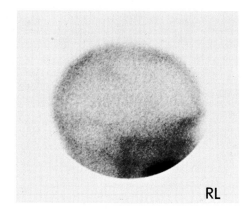

RL

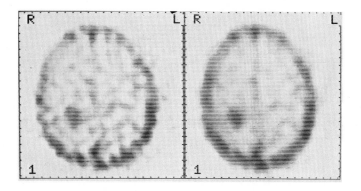

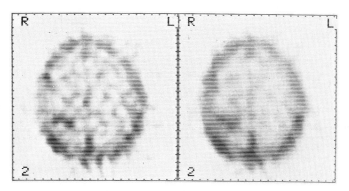

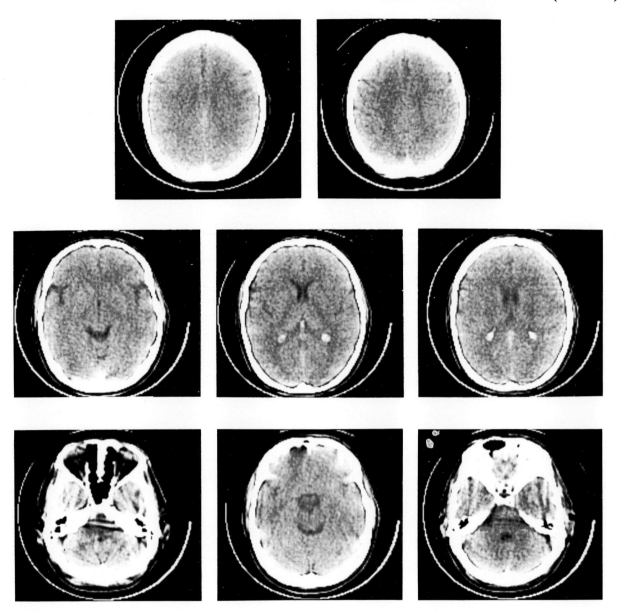

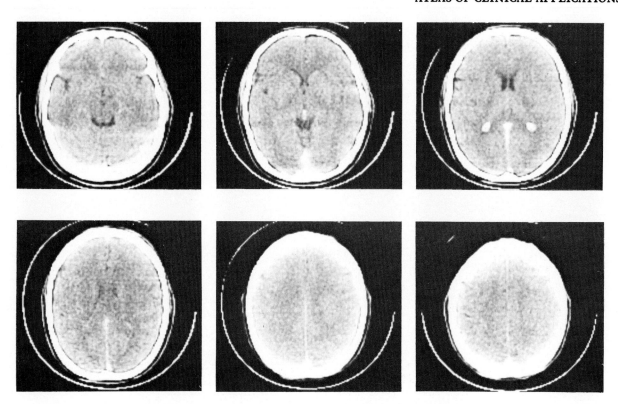

Patient 16

Clinical history	This 45-year-old man presented with a three month history of occipital headaches and vomiting. His memory had become impaired, especially during the previous four weeks. His wife had noticed a change in his personality.
On examination	There was a left sided hemiparesis with an extensor plantar response.

Provisional diagnosis. Cerebral tumour.

Imaging

Brain scan showed a round area of increased uptake in the right frontal region.

CET scan. There was a small area of greatly increased uptake in the right frontal region, close to the floor of the anterior fossa, which was surrounded by a halo of more diffuse uptake extending up into the right frontal lobe.

Right carotid angiogram showed a large right inferior frontal tumour, the upper part of which appeared avascular.

Outcome

At craniotomy, a small inferior right frontal glioma was found, associated with a large frontal cyst.

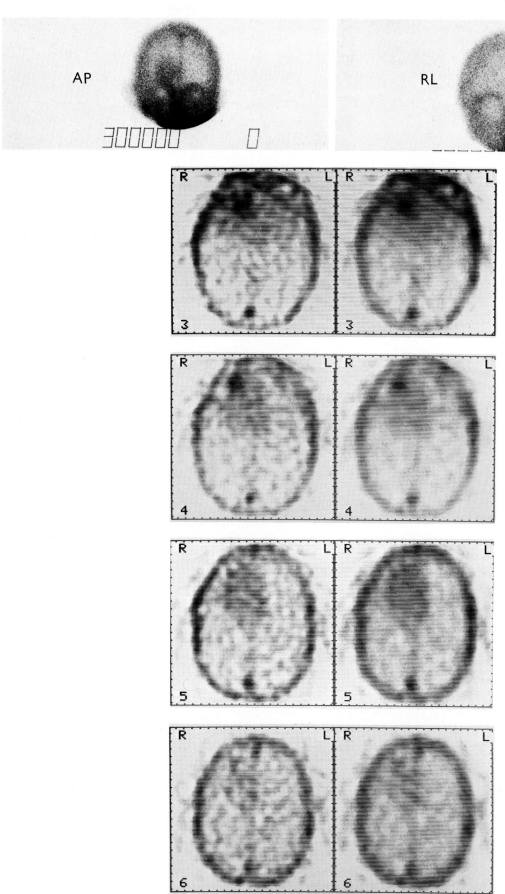

Patient 17

Clinical history

This 45-year-old female had a long history of right sided facial pain. Four years ago, bilateral carotid angiography was performed with negative outcome.

She was readmitted for investigation, with more intense right sided facial pain.

Imaging

Brain scan. Standard 4-view gamma camera scan appears normal: Dynamic perfusion sequence entirely normal.

CET scan. Tomograms of this patient show an area of increased uptake, round in shape, near to the mid-line and in the proximity of the right petrous apex.

Outcome

At operation, a right sided syncitial petrous apex meningioma was found.

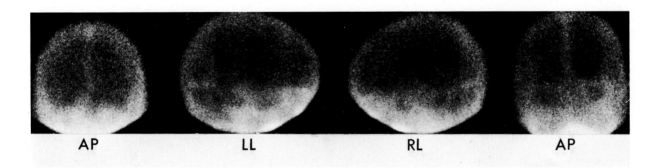

AP   LL   RL   AP

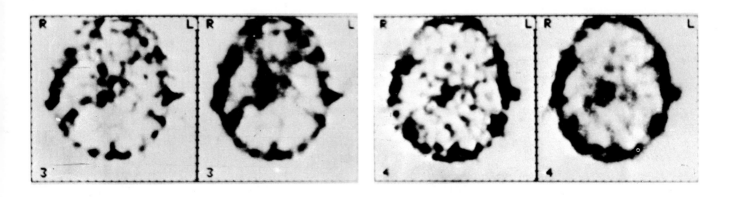

Patient 18

Clinical history

This 5½-year-old boy was referred with hydrocephalus. His birth had been normal and he had been well until eight weeks prior to admission when his mother noticed facial swelling and enlargement of his head. The child was less active than usual, he complained of headache when he cried and had a poor appetite.

On examination

The head was obviously enlarged; there was bilateral papilloedema, a right sided inferior temporal quadrantinopia, bilateral extensor plantar responses and ankle clonus.

Provisional diagnosis. Hydrocephalus of unknown cause.

Imaging

Brain scan. This showed a rounded area of increased activity in the suprasellar region to the left of the mid-line.

CET scan confirmed the presence of a mid-line lesion, extending to the left anteriorly, but also extending posteriorly to the region of the third ventricle.

4 Vessel angiography showed a mass with a capillary blush in the third ventricle, extending into the left lateral ventricle, supplied by the medial choroidal arteries.

Outcome

At craniotomy, a choroid plexus papilloma was removed, which arose in the 3rd ventricle and extended to the frontal horn of the left lateral ventricle.

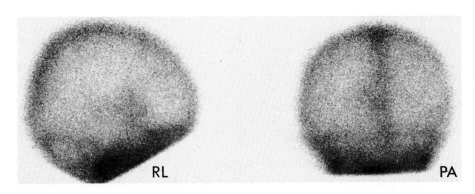

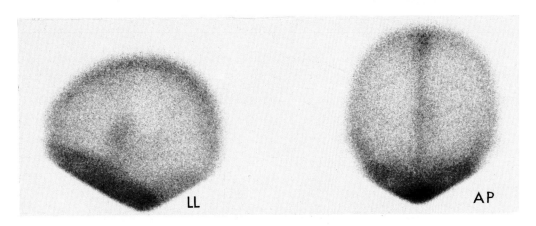

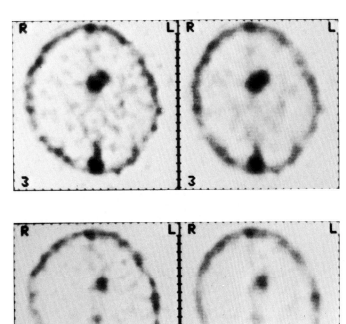

Patient 19

Clinical history

This 43-year-old man was admitted following three grand mal fits. Three weeks prior to admission, he had had a viral illness, accompanied by headaches, flashing lights and slight confusion. There had been a change in his personality since this illness. There were no abnormal physical signs.

Provisional diagnosis. Possible encephalitis.

Imaging

CET scan showed a rounded area of abnormal activity in the right parieto-occipital region, characteristic of a tumour.

CTT scan showed the lesion to be of mixed attenuation, and to show enhancement, compatible with either a tumour or leuko-encephalopathy.

Outcome

A right posterior parietal glioblastoma was partially removed at craniotomy.

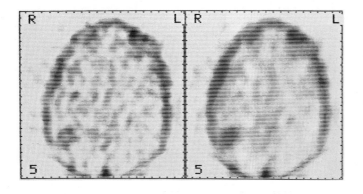

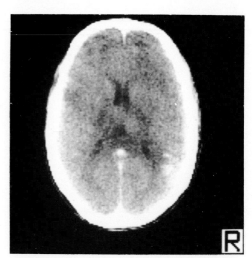

Patient 20

Clinical history

This 36-year-old woman had a history of a right parotid cylindroma excised ten years previously. Over the last five years, there had been several local recurrences of the tumour treated by excision, and there was also a large, slow-growing pulmonary metastasis.

Chemotherapy was instituted one year prior to this admission, which was precipitated by severe pain behind the right eye and in the right temporal region.

On examination

The patient was deaf in the right ear, and there was bilateral chronic papilloedema.

Provisional diagnosis. Cerebral metastases.

Imaging

Gamma camera brain scan. There is a large area of increased activity in the right temporal region.

CET scan confirmed the presence of abnormal activity involving the floor of the right middle fossa and extending superiorly into the right temporal lobe.

CTT scan showed a soft tissue mass in the right parotid region. The mass extended into the base of the skull and there were high attenuation areas in the right temporal lobe.

Final diagnosis

Extensive local recurrence of tumour with involvement of skull base and right temporal lobe.

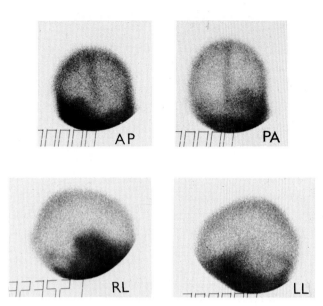

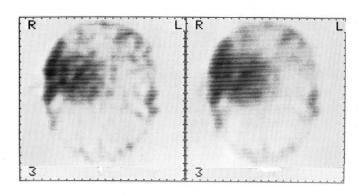

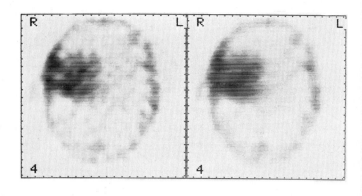

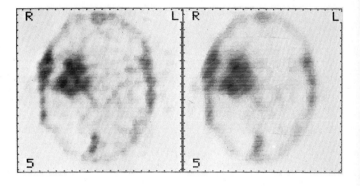

Patient 21

Clinical history

This 56-year-old man was admitted to hospital complaining of chest pain. The pain had been of sudden onset, 24 hours before and was crushing in nature, associated with sweating and nausea. Five days later, while still under investigation for this chest pain, he developed a sudden change in personality and became aggressive, uninhibited, confused and disorientated. On further questioning, his wife revealed that the patient had suffered frontal headaches for the previous month. All ECG's were normal and there was no biochemical evidence of myocardial damage.

On examination

There were no abnormal signs in the cardiovascular system. There was a left quadrantic homonymous field defect, fine nystagmus to the right and left, an ataxic gait, mild left hemiparesis, positive pout and snout reflexes, brisk tendon reflexes on the left, and a left sided extensor plantar response.

Provisional diagnosis. Possible right frontal tumour.

Imaging

CET scan showed extensive increased uptake in the right frontal lobe, which appeared to have a 'doughnut' configuration.

CTT scan showed a large cystic tumour in the right frontal region.

Outcome

Craniotomy and right frontal lobectomy was performed. Histology showed the lesion to be a glioblastoma multiforme (cystic astrocytoma grade IV).

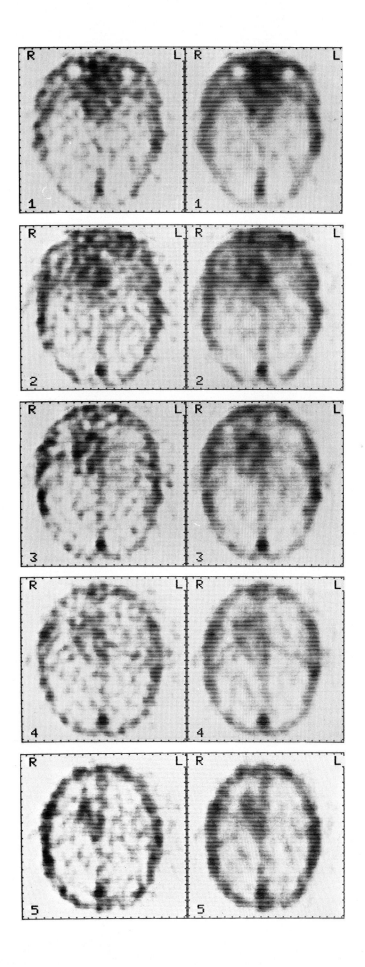

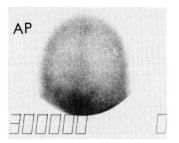

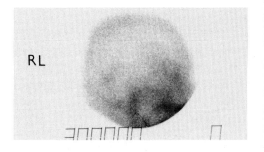

Patient 22

Clinical history

This 50-year-old woman had a four month history of frequent blackouts, thought to be epileptiform in nature. For two weeks prior to admission, she had become increasingly drowsy and had been vomiting.

On examination

She was drowsy and uncooperative. There was papilloedema of the right disc, left homonymous hemianopia, the left pupil was dilated, there was nystagmus to the right, a left facial weakness and left hemiparesis.

Provisional diagnosis. Cerebral tumour.

Imaging

Gamma camera brain scan was unhelpful.

CET scan showed a large area of increased activity in the right parietal lobe.

CTT scan showed a mass in the right parietal region which enhanced with contrast and was surrounded by oedema.

Outcome

A right parietal craniotomy was performed with subtotal evacuation of the tumour. Histology showed the lesion to be a grade II–III fibrillary astrocytoma.

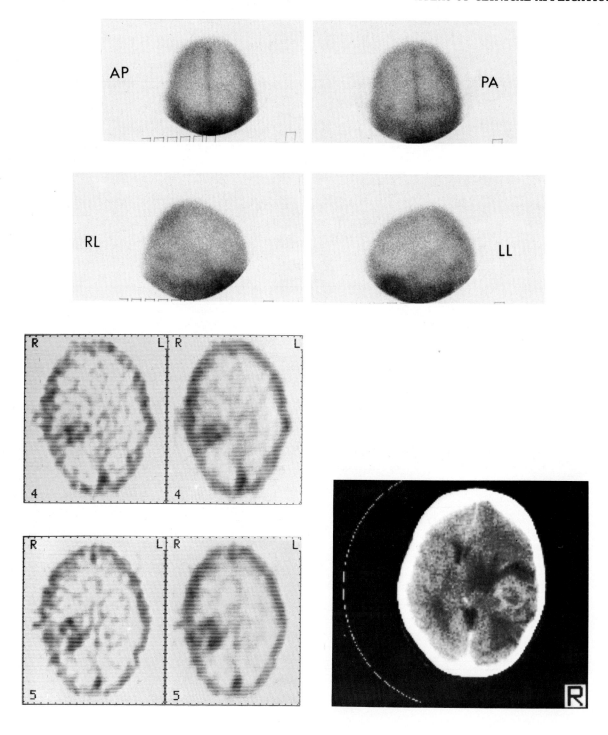

Patient 23

Clinical history

This 30-year-old woman was admitted with severe chronic bilateral papilloedema. Six months previously, she had been involved in a road traffic accident in which she sustained a head injury. Recently, she had developed episodes of bilateral obscuration of vision, and the papilloedema was discovered.

On examination

There was a mild left faciobrachial weakness.

Provisional diagnosis. Chronic subdural haematoma.

Imaging

Brain scan. The dynamic study showed a well defined area of abnormal activity, occurring in the capillary and venous phases, in the right temporal region.

Static gamma camera views confirmed the presence of a round lesion in the right temporal region.

CET scan showed the lesion to be peripheral extending up into the parietal region. It appeared to be characteristic of a meningioma, not of subdural.

CTT showed an enhancing lesion as above.

Outcome

On further questioning, the patient gave a history of periodic severe occipital headaches, which predated her head injury. A right convexity meningioma was completely removed, and the patient made a good recovery.

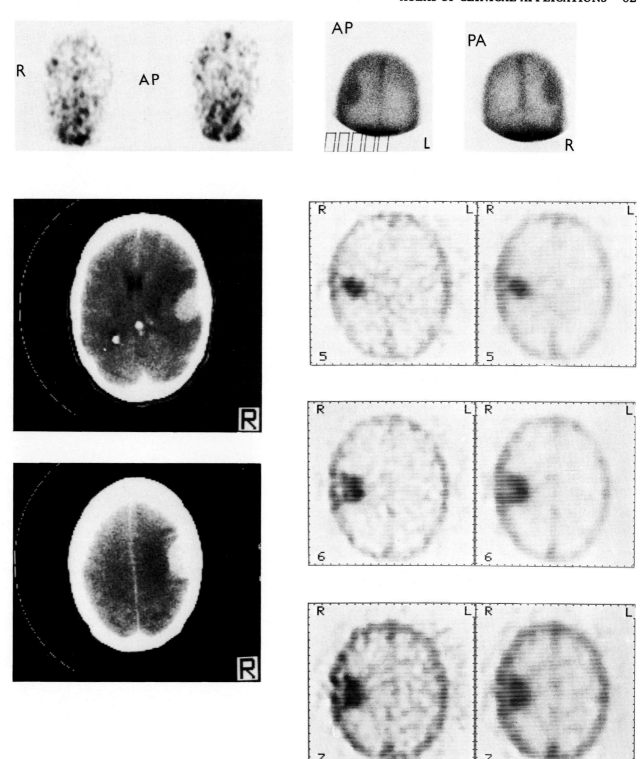

Patient 24

Clinical history   This 46-year-old woman gave a three month history of itching of the left eyelid. She had noticed the appearance of small black marks inside her lower lid and on the iris, and occasional blurring of vision in the left eye.

On examination   A brown tumour was visible through the left pupil and there were brown lesions inside the lower lid and on the inferior part of the iris.

Provisional diagnosis. Malignant melanoma with extrascleral extension. The left eye was enucleated.

Imaging   *CET scan* was performed 24 hours later and it showed increased activity in the left orbit, at the site of the recent surgery due to blood pooling. There was no evidence of metastatic disease.

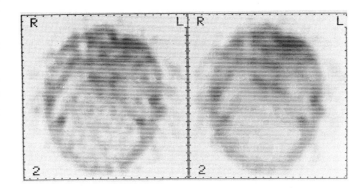

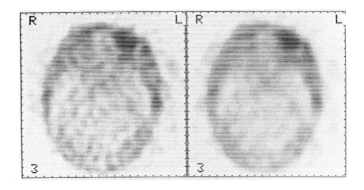

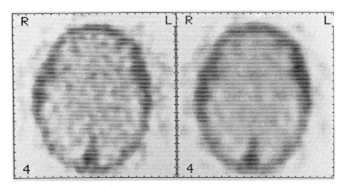

Patient 25

Clinical history This 64-year-old man presented with a six week history of personality change and occasional episodes of confusion. For one week, he had complained of right sided and occipital headaches, drowsiness and vomiting. His wife noticed that he dragged his left leg on walking.

On examination There was bilateral papilloedema, left sided hemiparesis and bilateral extensor plantar responses.

Provisional diagnosis. Right temporoparietal tumour.

Imaging *Skull X-ray* showed abnormal calcification in the region of the right temporal lobe.

CET scan showed a round area of increased activity in the right temporoparietal region.

CTT scan showed a high attenuation area in the right temporal region.

Outcome A partial right temporal lobectomy was performed. Histology showed the lesion to be a grade II-III fibrillary astrocytoma with oligodendroglial components and extensive calcification.

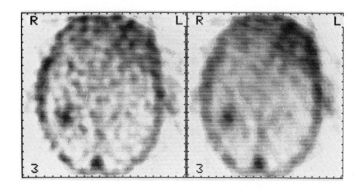

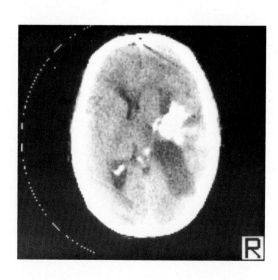

Patient 26

Clinical history

This 53-year-old woman had had an episode of loss of consciousness two months prior to admission, and since then had complained of odd sensations in the left side of her body, like water trickling down from her waist to her toes. For four weeks, she had complained of numbness of the left hand, and had developed a left facial nerve palsy.

On examination

There was complete left hemianaesthesia, and global weakness of the left arm, and a left upper motor neurone facial nerve palsy.

Provisional diagnosis. Cerebral tumour.

Imaging

Gamma camera brain scan showed a large round area of increased activity in the right parietal region.

CET scan. The tomograms confirmed the lesion. One slice showed the lesion to have a cold centre or doughnut configuration.

CTT scan showed a large mass of mixed attenuation in the right parietal region, which enhanced and showed probable necrosis.

Outcome

At craniotomy, a large glioma was partially excised. Histology showed a grade III astrocytoma.

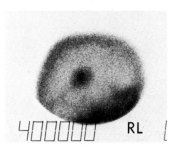

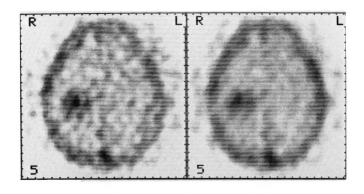

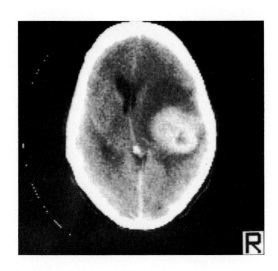

Patient 27

Clinical history

This 43-year-old man complained of two transient (10 second) episodes of blindness in his right eye, accompanied by loss of speech and numbness of the right side of his tongue. On questioning, he gave a four month history of occipital headaches, but was otherwise well. In the past, he had suffered from migrainous headaches, often preceded by tunnel vision.

On examination

There was a mild left proptosis, bilateral anosmia, bilateral papilloedema, the right tendon reflexes were increased and there were bilateral extensor plantar responses.

Skull X-ray had shown thickening of the left wing of the sphenoid with abnormal calcification in the left frontal region, and erosion of the dorsum sellae.

Provisional diagnosis. Probable frontal meningioma.

Imaging

Brain scan. This showed a large area of increased activity in the left frontal region.

CET scan confirmed the abnormality, which involved the floor of the left anterior fossa, extending upwards into the left frontal lobe and reaching the mid-line.

CTT scan showed a large high attenuation lesion in the same position.

Left carotid angiogram showed a large frontal meningioma with subfalcine herniation.

Outcome

At craniotomy, a large left frontal convexity meningioma was removed.

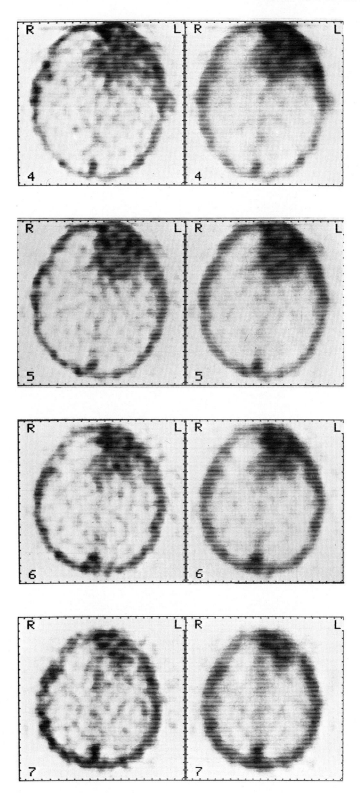

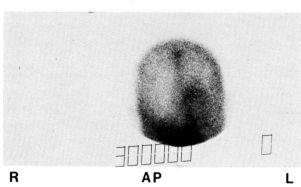

LL   R   AP   L

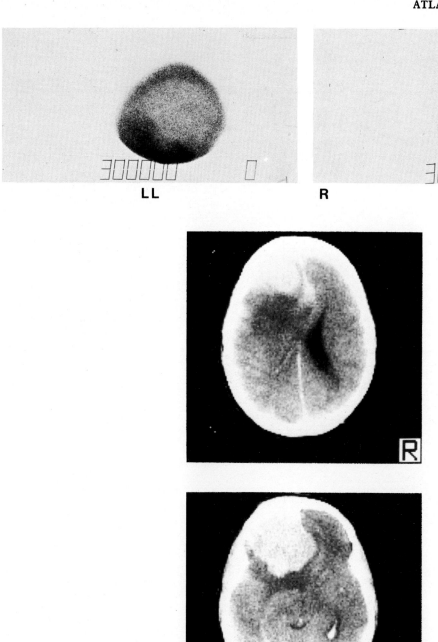

Patient 28

Clinical history	This 64-year-old woman had developed sudden vertigo and deafness in the left ear one year prior to admission. She had recently complained of unsteady gait, with frequent falls, diplopia on right lateral gaze, and occipital headaches.
On examination	There was first degree nystagmus to the right, vertical nystagmus, diplopia, left sided sensory Vth nerve palsy with absent corneal reflex, mild left VIIth nerve palsy, complete deafness on the left and a positive Romberg sign.
	Provisional diagnosis. Left sided cerebello-pontine angle tumour, probable acoustic neuroma.
Imaging	*Brain scan* showed a round area of increased activity in the region of the left cerebello-pontine angle.
	CET scan confirmed this lesion to be in the region of the left petrous apex.
	CTT scan showed a round enhancing low density lesion at the left cerebello-pontine angle.
Outcome	An acoustic neuroma was removed at craniotomy.

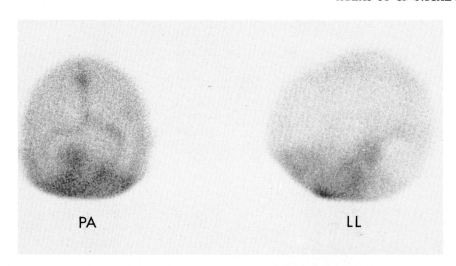

PA   LL

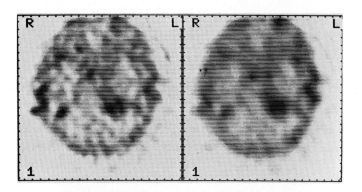

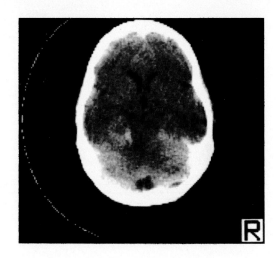

Patient 29

Clinical history   This 70-year-old man had a two year history of grand mal epilepsy, for which no cause was originally found. He now presented with a right sided weakness and dysphasia.

Provisional diagnosis. Possible cerebral tumour.

Imaging   *CET scan* showed a large round area of increased activity in the left parietal lobe.

CTT scan confirmed the lesion, which was of low density and showed some enhancement after contrast.

Final diagnosis   Right parietal tumour.

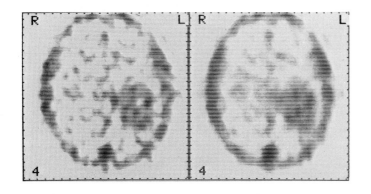

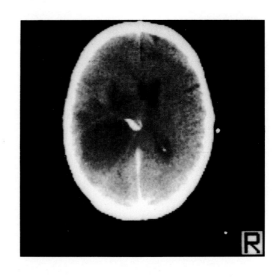

Patient 30

Clinical history

This 48-year-old man had originally presented three years ago with right temporal lobe epilepsy. He was subsequently found to have a right temporal lobe tumour, which was removed at craniotomy. Histology showed a glioblastoma multiforme. He had remained well since.

He was admitted, complaining of weakness and numbness of the left side of his body, a tendency to fall to the left and an unsteady gait.

Imaging

Gamma camera brain scan showed increased activity in the temporoparietal region.

CET scan confirmed this abnormality and showed the lesion to extend to the mid-line.

CTT scan showed a low attenuation area in the right temporal region, but medial to it was a mass which enhanced with contrast.

Final diagnosis

Recurrent glioblastoma multiforme.

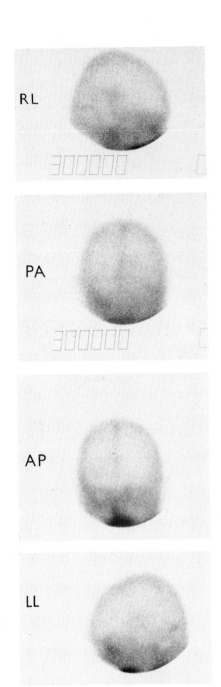

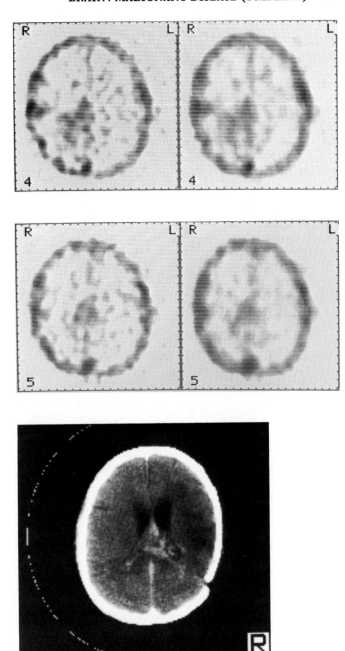

Patient 31

Clinical history

This 66-year-old man originally presented one year prior to this admission, complaining of unsteady gait, and falling to the left. At that time, he had left sided V[th] and VIIth nerve palsies, and ataxia. CTT scan at that time showed hydrocephalus and a ventricular shunt was inserted with good effect. However, over the next few months, the patient's condition deteriorated, with severely ataxic gait, weakness of both legs, slurred speech and a palatal palsy.

Imaging

4 vessel angiography showed a large meningioma in the left cerebello-pontine angle, extending supra and infra-tentorially. This finding was confirmed on the CTT scan.

Brain scan showed increased uptake in the left cerebello-pontine angle region. *CET scan* showed this to extend forwards into the middle fossa.

Final diagnosis

Large cerebello-pontine angle meningioma, extending supratentorially.

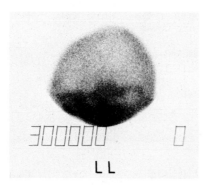

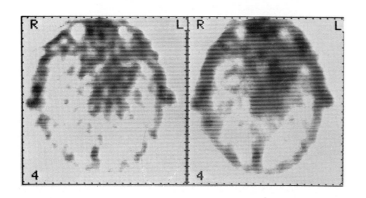

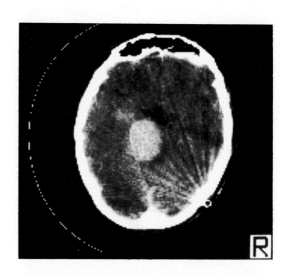

Brain: malignant disease (secondary)

Patient 32

Clinical history This 66-year-old woman was known to have metastatic carcinoma of the breast. She was admitted complaining of severe pain in the right temporal region and right side of her face, and was thought to show some personality change.

    Skull X-ray showed several lytic metastases.

Provisional diagnosis. Possible cerebral metastases.

Imaging *Brain scan.* The dynamic study showed a marked blush of activity in the right parietal region which appeared in the capillary phase and persisted to the venous phase.

CET scan showed a round area of increased activity lying high in the right parietal region. Although this lesion was peripheral, it appeared to extend into the right cerebral hemisphere, and was characteristic of a very vascular tumour, either a meningioma or secondary deposit.

Outcome Biopsy of the lesion via a burrhole was carried out, and a large vascular metastasis was discovered which arose in the skull but involved the meninges.

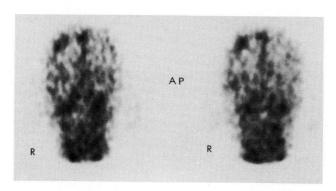

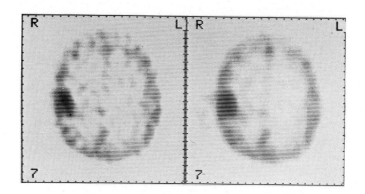

Patient 33

Clinical history
This 72-year-old man complained of a single episode of transient right sided weakness, and confusion. His symptoms had resolved rapidly and there were no abnormal physical signs on examination. He had a four month history of carcinoma of the bronchus, for which he was receiving chemotherapy.

Provisional diagnosis. Transient ischaemic attack; possible cerebral metastases.

Imaging
Gamma camera brain scan showed a single large round area of increased activity in the left parieto-occipital region, compatible with a cerebral tumour.

CET scan. The section scan improves depth localization of this lesion.

Final diagnosis
Cerebral metastasis from carcinoma of the bronchus.

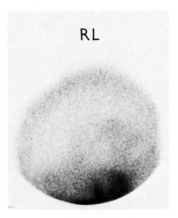

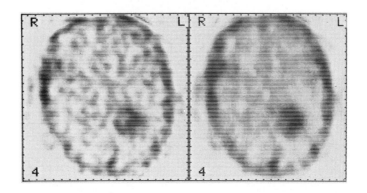

Patient 34

Clinical history   This female patient, aged 50 years, with a 4 year history of carcinoma of the left breast, presented with a recent episode of focal epilepsy.

Imaging   *Gamma camera brain scan. A single* abnormality is seen in the static 4-view study (left frontal area).

CET scan. Two lesions are shown: one in the left frontal lobe, and another in the right parietal lobe deep in the substance of the brain, close to the mid-line.

Outcome   A diagnosis of multiple brain secondaries can now be made.

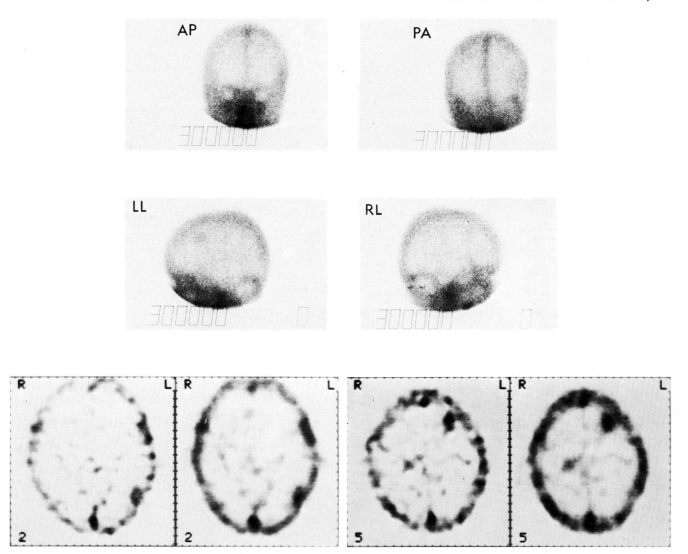

Patient 35

Clinical history   52-year-old female, who had a breast carcinoma removed five years ago, presented with persistent headaches, right sided papilloedema and vomiting.

Provisional diagnosis. Cerebral secondaries.

Imaging   *Brain scan.* Gamma camera studies showed multiple areas of abnormal uptake. *Differential Diagnosis.* ? brain or skull secondaries.

CET scan shows multiple intracerebral lesions.

Final diagnosis   Multiple cerebral metastases.

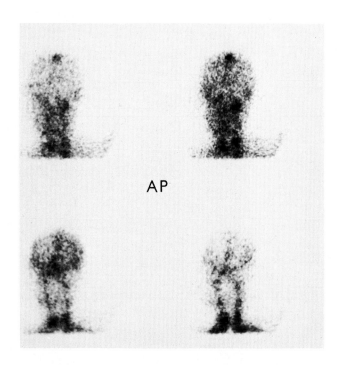

AP

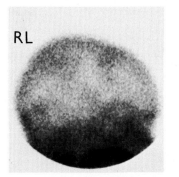

RL

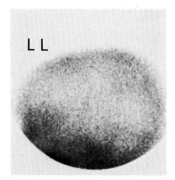

L L

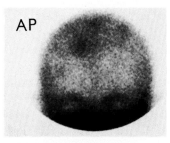

AP

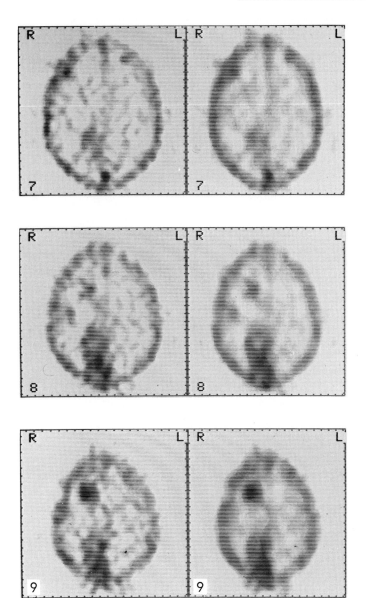

Patient 36

Clinical history This 66-year-old man had undergone thoracotomy and left upper lobectomy one year previously for adenocarcinoma of the bronchus. He was readmitted with a mild left sided weakness and truncal ataxia.

Provisional diagnosis. Cerebral metastases.

Imaging *CET scan.* There are multiple areas of increased activity in the left parietal and frontal lobes and right temporal lobe (slices 5 and 6) and left and right fronto-parietal regions at a higher level.

Final diagnosis Multiple cerebral metastases were confirmed.

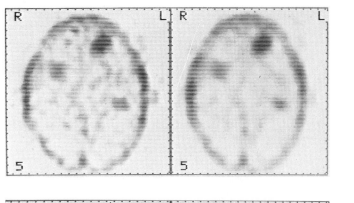

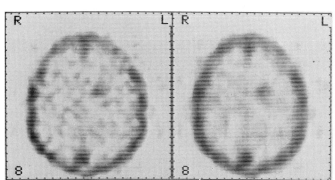

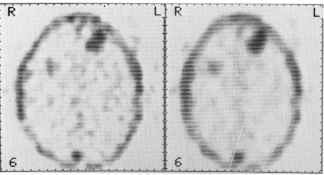

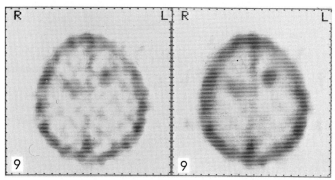

Patient 37

Clinical history	This 67-year-old man was admitted after an episode of numbness and twitching of his right hand, followed by twitching of the right side of his face. On questioning, he admitted to two similar previous fits in the past four months. He gave a history of ischaemic heart disease with angina pectoris, and he had smoked 5 cigarettes per day for many years.
On examination	There was a mild pyramidal weakness of the right upper limb.
	Chest X-ray showed a mass in the right mid zone in the anterior segment of the right upper lobe.
	Provisional diagnosis. Carcinoma of bronchus with cerebral metastases.
Imaging	*Gamma camera brain scan. This was unhelpful*—no well defined lesions were seen.
	CET scan showed three well defined round areas of increased activity in the right posterior parietal lobe, the right frontal lobe, and the left parietal lobe, compatible with the presence of cerebral metastases.
	CTT scan showed the same three lesions, as areas of increased attenuation with some contrast enhancement.
Outcome	The pulmonary mass was biopsied and histology confirmed the presence of a squamous cell carcinoma.

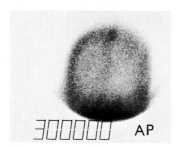

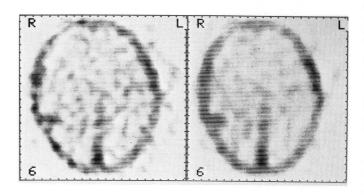

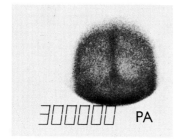

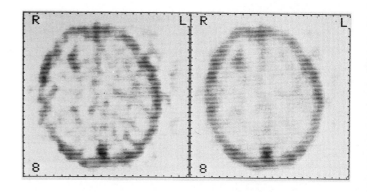

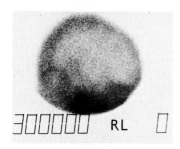

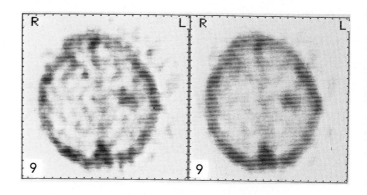

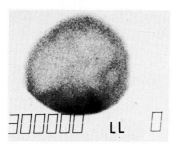

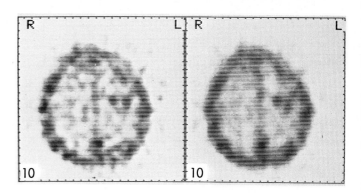

Patient 38

Diagnosis   60-year-old female with carcinoma of right breast.

Imaging   *CET scan.* Multiple cerebral secondaries are seen.

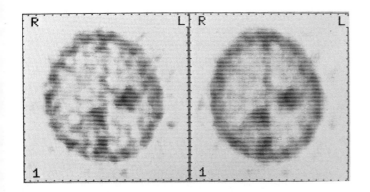

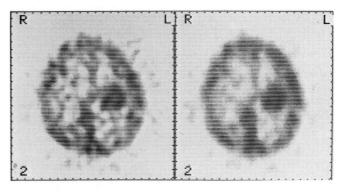

Patient 39

Diagnosis   Carcinoma of the breast. 50-year-old female presenting with focal
                   neurological signs and symptoms.

Imaging   *CET scan* confirms multiple cerebral secondaries—left frontal, right parietal,
                   right occipital, possibly also right temporal and left parietal.

Outcome   Cerebral secondaries from breast carcinoma.

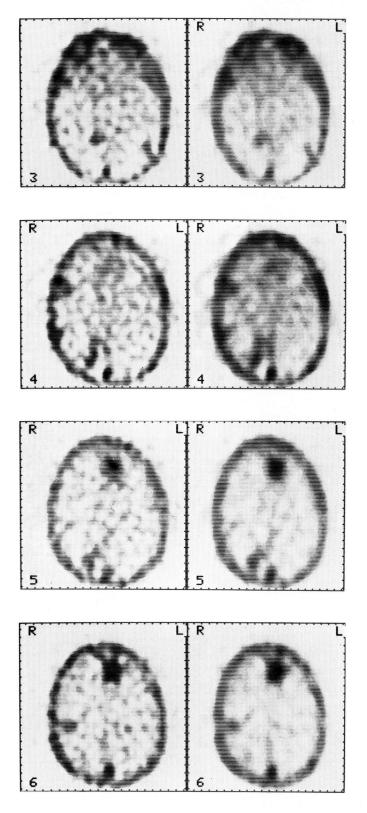

Patient 40

Clinical history	This female patient, aged 67 years, had a 6 year history of carcinoma of the breast. Previous investigations had revealed bony secondaries in the cervical spine. She recently presented with diplopia to the right and a right sixth nerve palsy.
Imaging	*Brain scan.* Multiple areas of increased and abnormal tracer uptake are seen. It is, however, difficult to decide the extent of intracerebral involvement.
	CET scan. Emission tomography shows all the lesions to be in the skull.
Final diagnosis	Skull secondaries. No evidence of brain secondaries.

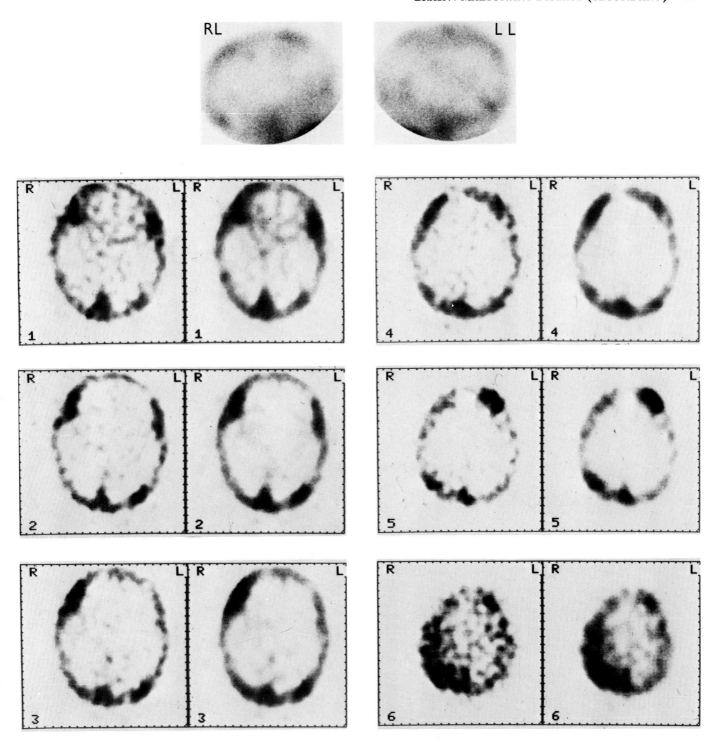

Patient 41

Diagnosis	Female patient, aged 57 years, referred for routine brain scan following removal of malignant melanoma of the right ear.
Imaging	*Gamma camera brain scan,* an area of diffuse increased tracer uptake is seen in a posterior location, on the right side.
	CET scan. The significance and exact extent of this is seen on the section scan. The abnormal uptake is confined to the scalp and skull, and is a consequence of the surgical intervention.
Outcome	No evidence of space occupying disease in the brain.

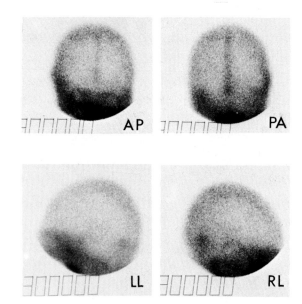

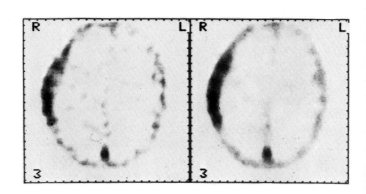

Bone imaging: skull

Patient 42

Diagnosis

43-year-old female patient with primary hyperparathyroidism.

Imaging

CET scan: skull tomograms. Note high resolution scan with a wealth of anatomical detail unobtainable with conventional two-dimensional imaging.

The increased contrast resolution is partly a consequence of the underlying physiology, i.e., hypercalcaemia, and increased uptake of the bone seeking radiopharmaceutical (improved signal/noise ratio).

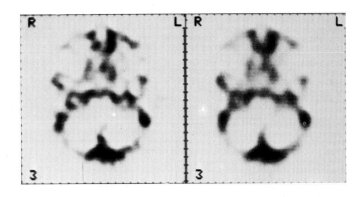

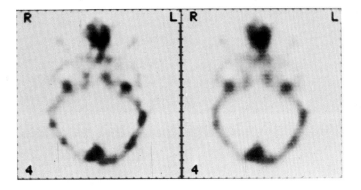

Patient 43

Clinical history

This female patient, aged 40 years, had a carcinoma of the right breast diagnosed one year ago. She now presented with skin nodules, severe pain on the left side of the bridge of the nose, the thoracic spine and right shoulder.

Imaging

Whole body bone scan. This scan is essentially within normal limits.

CET scan (skull). Surprisingly, the tomogram reveals a large space occupying lesion of unknown origin in the left occipital lobe which concentrates ^{99m}Tc-MDP. Several tomographic slices do not show involvement of nasal bones.

CET scan (brain). The tomograms with standard ^{99m}Tc-pertechnetate confirm a large left occipital lobe lesion with a possible second lesion anteriorly.

Outcome

Cerebral secondaries.

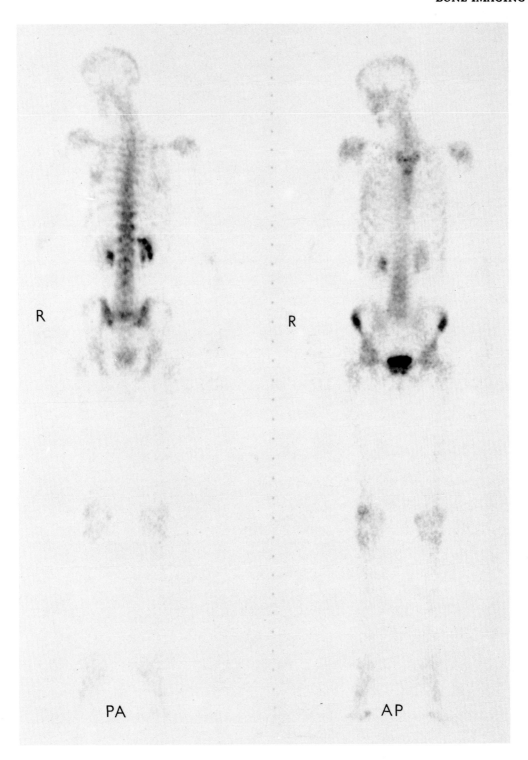

R

R

PA

AP

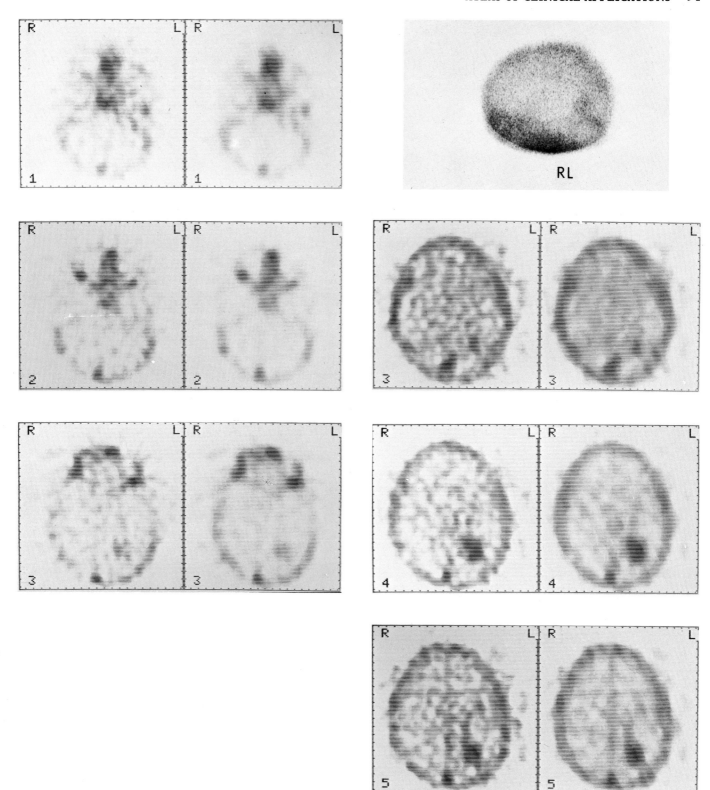

Patient 44

Clinical history	This 40-year-old patient presented one year ago with carcinoma of the right breast which was surgically removed. On referral, there was pain and proptosis of the right eye.
Imaging	*Whole body bone scan.* Increased abnormal tracer uptake was detected in the skull, but precise definition of its site and extent was difficult to assess. Multiple but small areas of asymmetric uptake were detected in several spinal processes. There was marked scoliosis.
	CET scan (skull). The tomographic slices allow clear definition of the extent of involvement: right orbit, frontal, temporal and parietal bones.
Final diagnosis	Multiple bony secondaries.

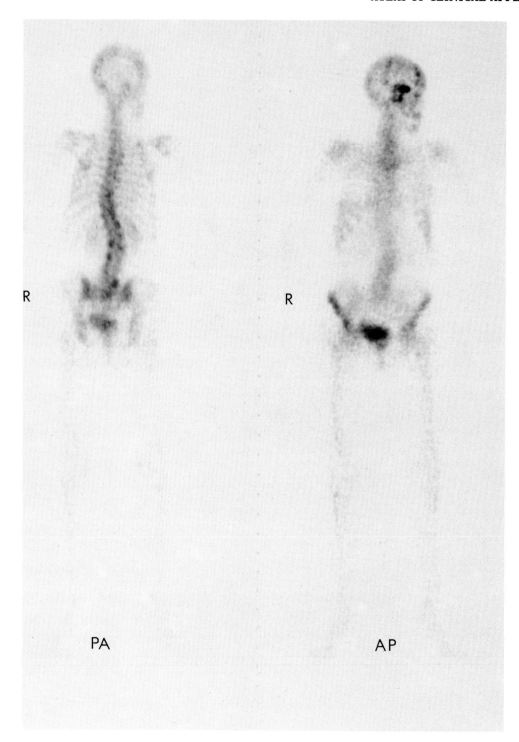

R

R

PA

AP

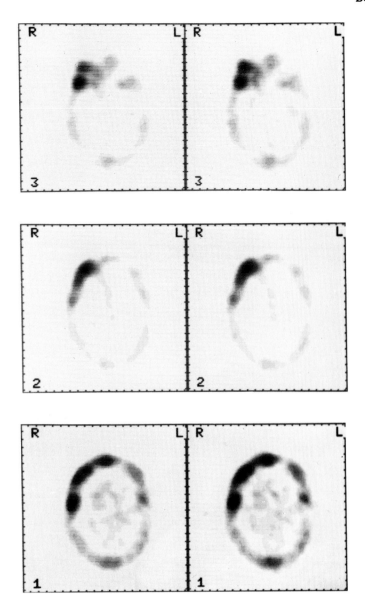

Patient 45

Diagnosis   Female patient with carcinoma of the breast.

Imaging   *Whole body bone scan.* The scan shows an area of increased uptake in the left parietal bone corresponding to the lesion seen on the lateral skull X-ray.

CET scan (skull). The section scan demonstrates the structural detail of the lesion, showing tracer uptake in front, and behind the main lesion, which metabolically is silent.

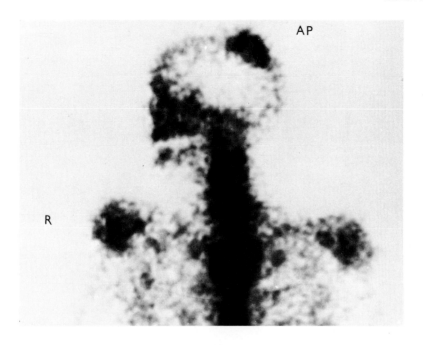

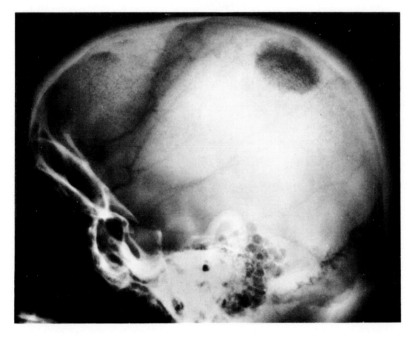

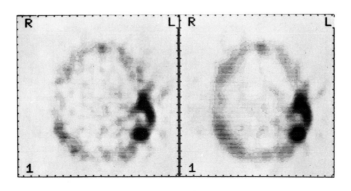

Patient 46

Diagnosis

60-year-old male with Paget's disease of bone.

Imaging

Whole body bone scan. Extensive tracer uptake in the skull, spine, sacroiliac joints and right shoulder.

CET scan (skull). Shows the pattern of tracer uptake within the two tables of the skull.

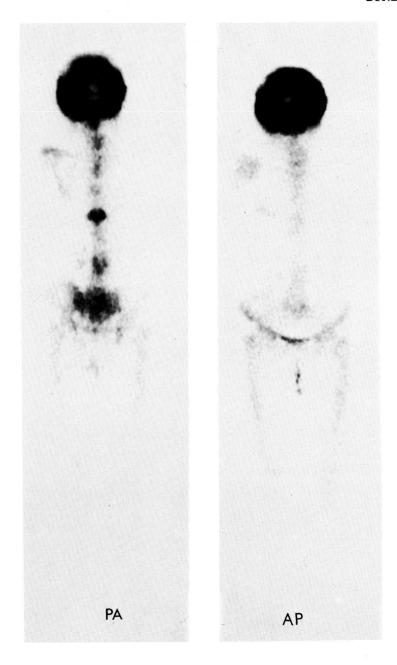

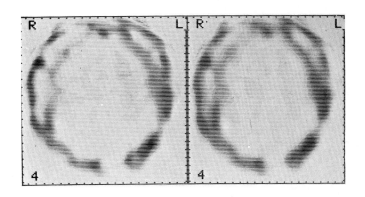

Patient 47

Diagnosis

45-year-old female with four year history of carcinoma of the left breast. Referred for follow-up bone scan.

Imaging

Whole body bone scan. Abnormal but ill-defined uptake in the skull and suspicious focal uptake in the costochondral joints and greater trochanter of the right femur.

CET scan (skull). Multiple and well defined areas of abnormal focal uptake confirm the presence of several bony secondaries.

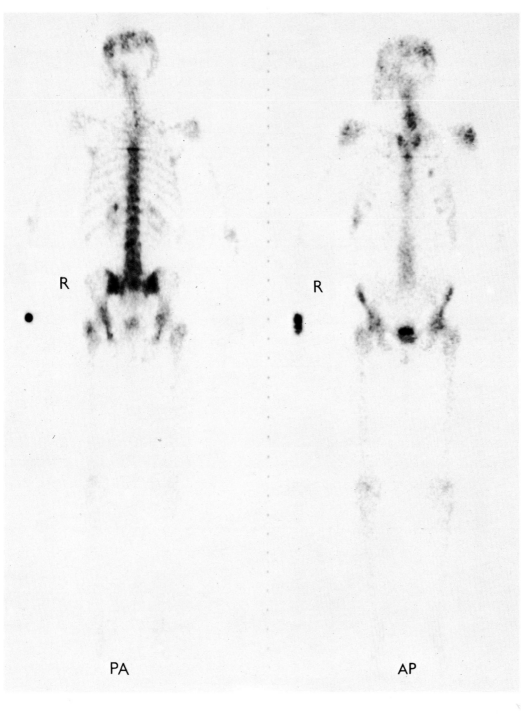

PA
AP

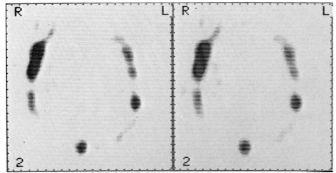
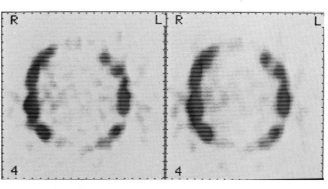

Patient 48

Diagnosis	50-year-old female with juxta-cortical osteosarcoma of the distal end of the right femur. Otherwise well. Normal chest X-ray.
Imaging	*Whole body bone scan.* An extensive area of abnormal tracer uptake is seen in the primary tumour. In addition, a doubtful area of focal uptake is seen in the left skull. For confirmation, spot gamma camera scans were obtained. The area of abnormal uptake is confirmed, probably in the left frontal bone.
	CET bone scan (skull). The relevant section scan reveals the real localization of the lesion—within the soft tissue of the left temple.
Outcome	*A 2.3 mm lesion* in *soft tissue* was removed and histology confirmed it to be a malignant secondary from the primary osteosarcoma. Two months later, a repeat whole body bone scan revealed *soft tissue lung secondaries*. At this time, chest X-ray was normal. Six weeks later, a new whole body bone scan confirmed rapid progression of soft tissue lung deposits. Chest X-ray confirmed these lesions.

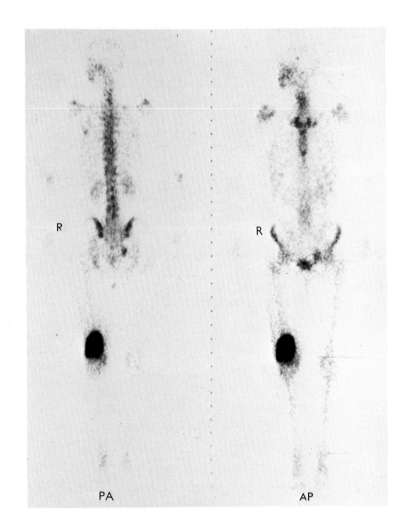

PA   AP

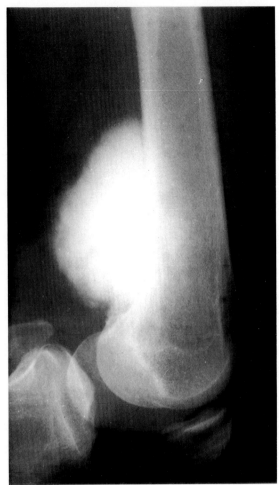

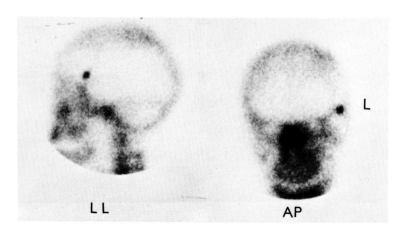

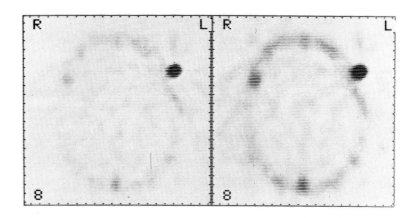

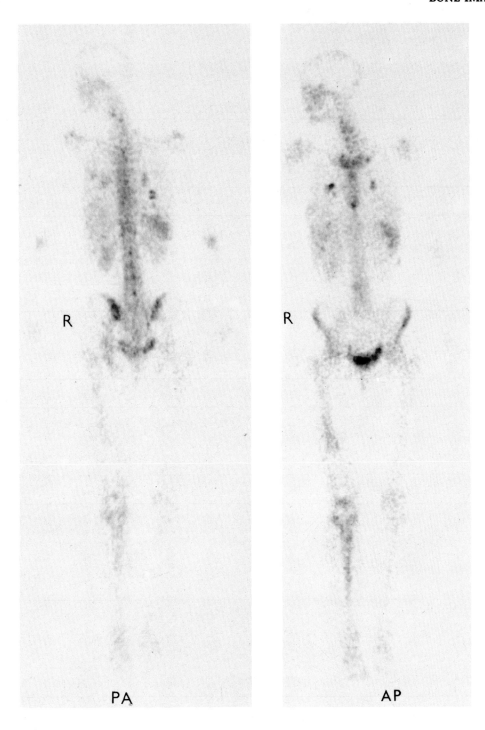

R

R

PA

AP

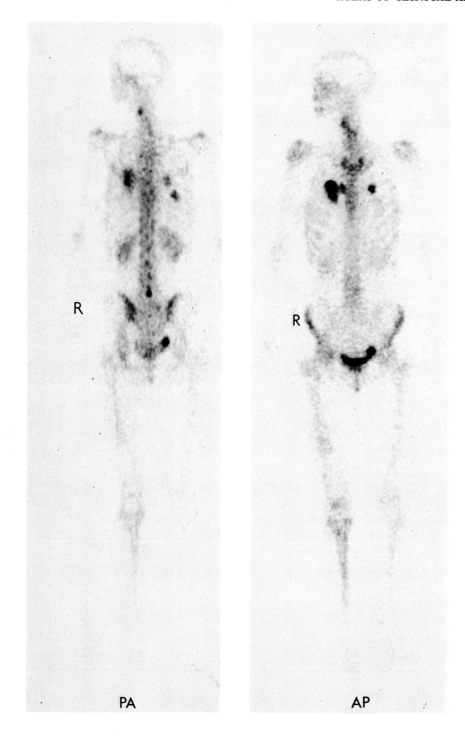

PA   AP

Patient 49

Clinical history   This 51-year-old female with carcinoma of the cervix presented with lumbar pain and was referred for a whole body bone scan.

Imaging   *Whole body bone scan.* A well defined single area of increased tracer uptake is seen in the frontal region of the skull.

CET scan (skull). The section scans confirm this abnormality to be a lesion in the left frontal bone.

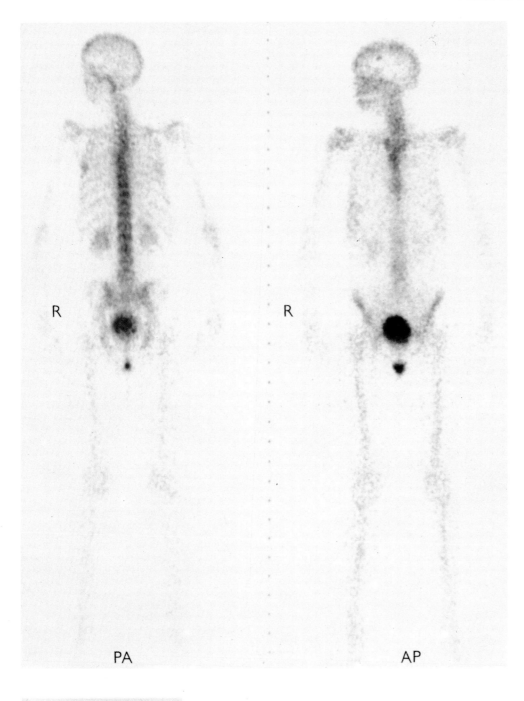

PA

R

AP

R

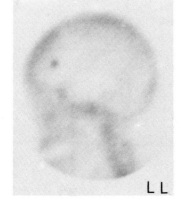

L L

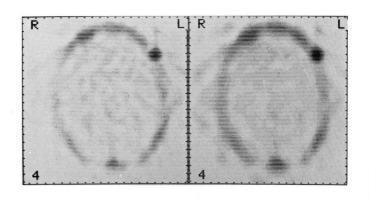

Patient 50

Diagnosis

56-year-old male with oat cell carcinoma of the bronchus

Imaging

Whole body bone scan. There is evidence of multiple skeletal secondaries involving the lower dorsal spine, mid lumbar spine, left sacroiliac joint and right ischium. The base of the skull is also involved.

CET scan (skull). Section scans reveal involvement of the left sphenoid bone and anterior fossa.

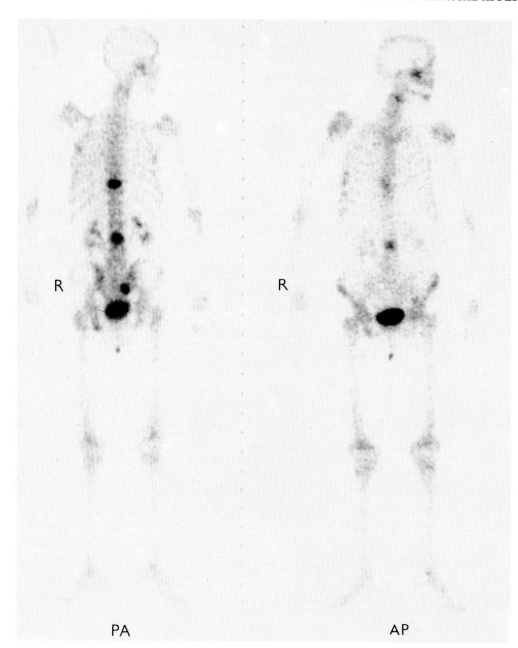

PA   AP

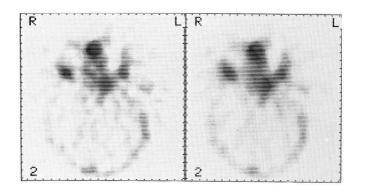

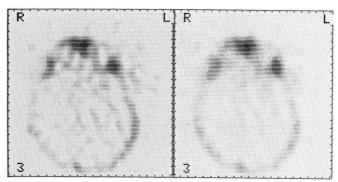

Patient 51

Clinical history   This 58-year-old male with squamous cell carcinoma of the right ear had a mastoidectomy performed six years ago. He was admitted with meningitis and pain over the site of the operation.

Imaging   *Whole body bone scan.* A single area of abnormal and focal tracer uptake is seen at the base of the skull. In addition, there is uptake in the right shoulder joint due to long-standing arthritis.

CET scan (skull). Abnormal tracer uptake is demonstrated, involving the right mastoid area, extending forward into the petrous bone. There is involvement of the left petrous bone and abnormal tracer concentration is seen within the left posterior fossa.

Conclusion   There is evidence of recurrence of the tumour. A CTT scan failed to resolve the question of the abnormality discovered in the left posterior fossa.

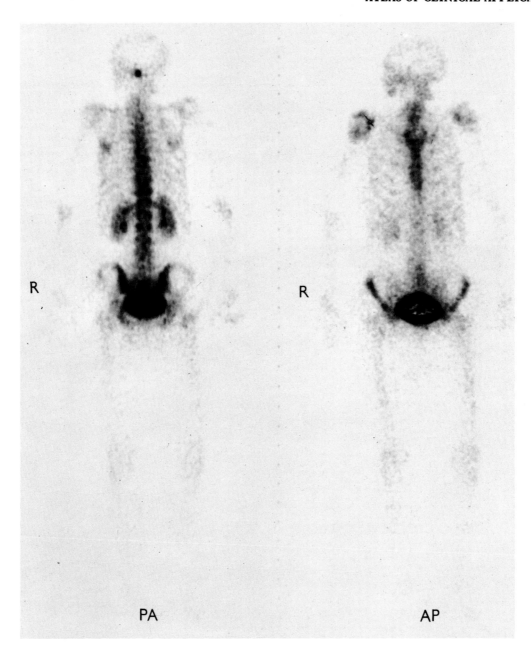

PA   AP

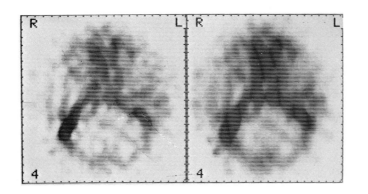

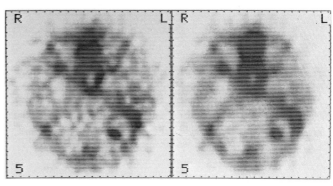

Bone imaging: chest and knees

Patient 52

Diagnosis
7-year-old boy with primary osteosarcoma of the right tibia.

Imaging
Whole body bone scan. Apart from tracer uptake within the tumour, no abnormalities were detected.

CET scan. Transverse section of the chest. Note resolution of spinal canal.

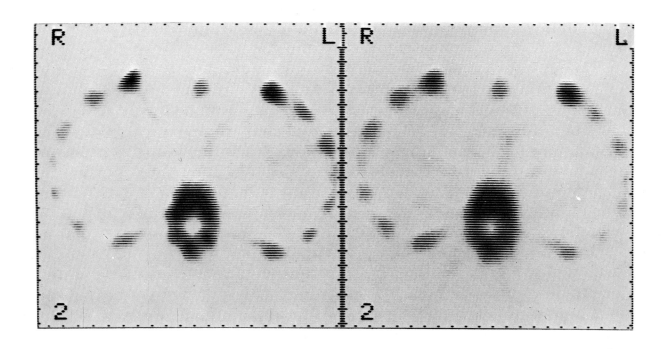

Patient 53

Diagnosis 7-year-old girl with Ewing's sarcoma of the right tibia.

Imaging *Whole body bone scan.* Features of a growing skeleton. Abnormal focal uptake in the upper two-thirds of the right tibia. No further evidence of skeletal involvement.

CET scan. Tomograms of the chest and the legs at the level of the proximal third of the tibia are shown. Abnormal tumour uptake is confirmed in the tomograms of the right tibia. Normal tracer distribution in the chest.

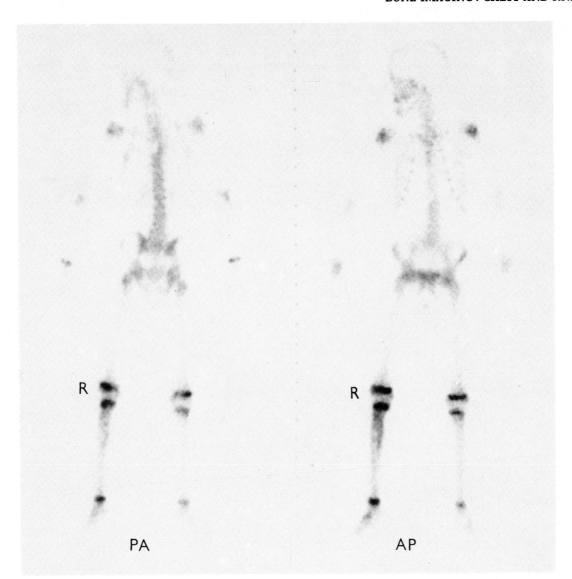

PA   AP

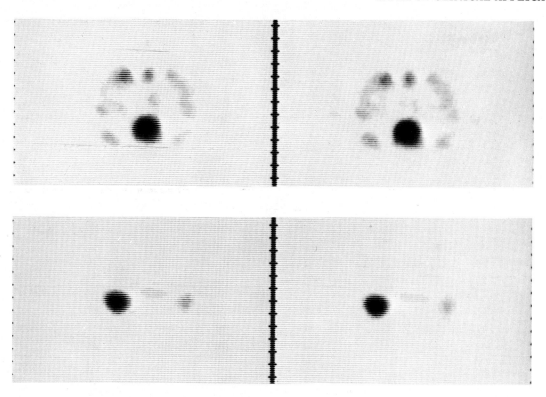

Patient 54

Diagnosis   14-year-old boy with primary osteosarcoma of the left femur. Amputation was performed and three months later a whole body bone scan was obtained.

Imaging   *Whole body bone scan and gamma camera scans.* Evidence of soft tissue uptake of the bone seeking radiopharmaceutical within the chest. Features of a growing skeleton.

CET scan. Confirms lesions within the soft tissue of the lungs.

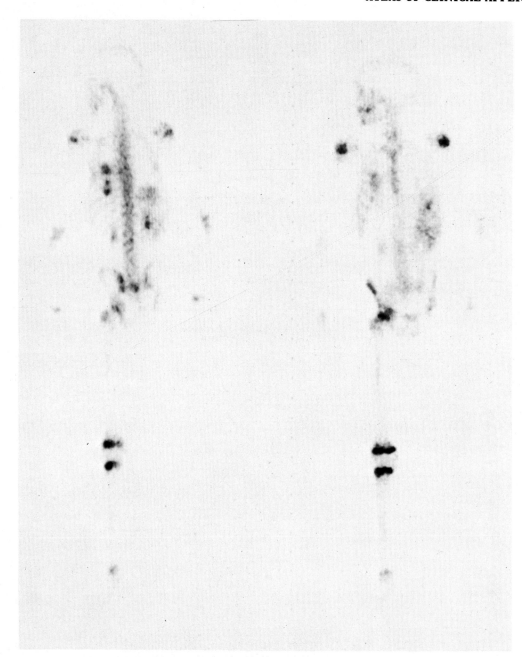

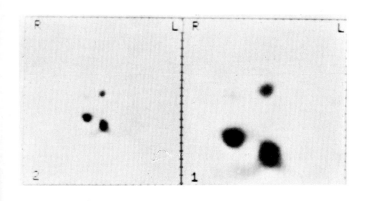

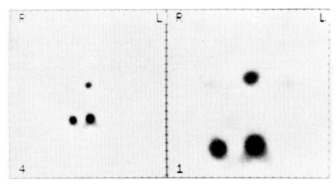

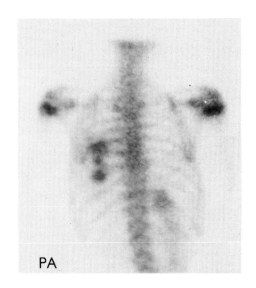

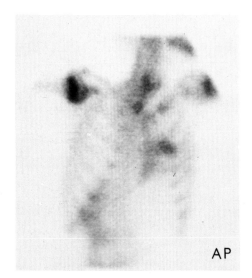

Patient 55

Clinical history

This 14-year-old boy complained of pain in both knees on exertion, with tenderness on forced extension. X-rays showed no abnormalities.

Imaging

Whole body bone scan. Features of a normal growing skeleton. Little uptake in either patella.

CET scan. Section scans confirms this to be the case. Note remarkable detail of the condyles. There is more information in this tomogram than there is in the two-dimensional standard gamma camera views.

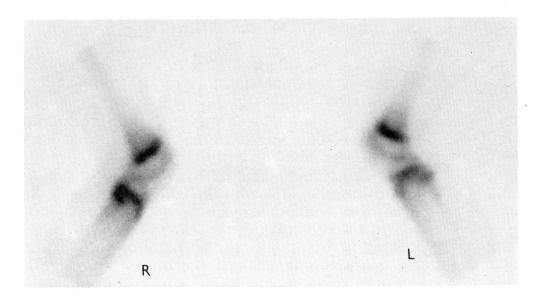

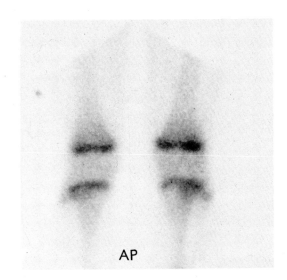

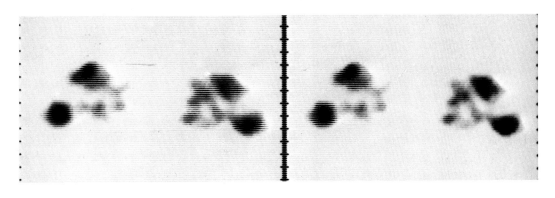

Liver and spleen

Patient 56

Diagnosis

67-year-old male with Hodgkin's disease. Referred for follow-up with a two month history of loin pain and a mass in the right iliac fossa.

Imaging

Gamma camera scan. Normal pattern of tracer distribution in the liver. No splenic tissue visualization (previous diagnostic splenectomy undertaken).

CET scan. Note pattern of normal tomograms of the liver. Care must be exercised in the analysis of liver tomograms.

Diagrams 1–7

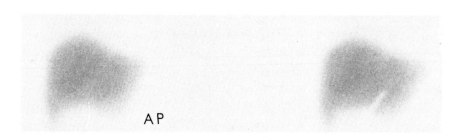

AP

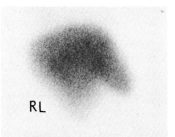

RL

PA

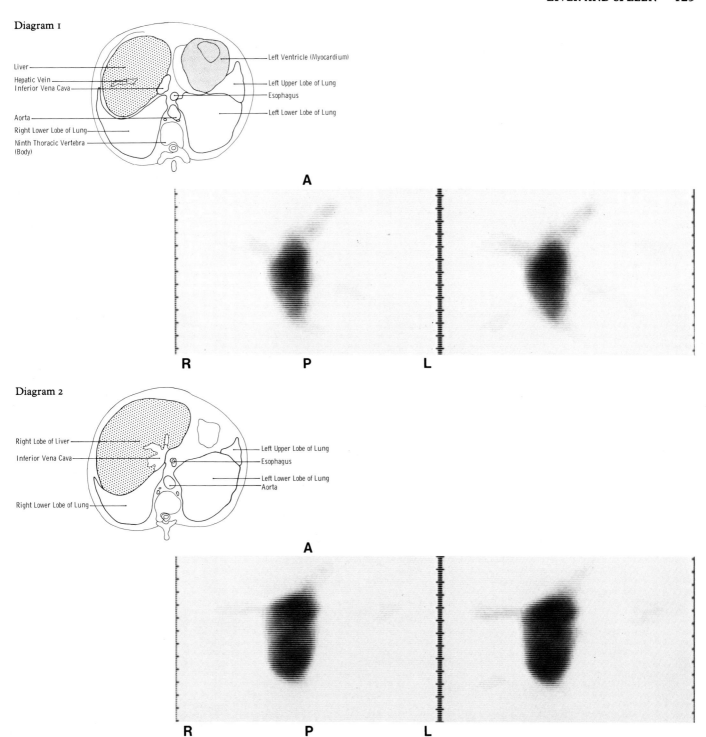

Diagram 1

Liver
Hepatic Vein
Inferior Vena Cava
Aorta
Right Lower Lobe of Lung
Ninth Thoracic Vertebra (Body)

Left Ventricle (Myocardium)
Left Upper Lobe of Lung
Esophagus
Left Lower Lobe of Lung

A

R   P   L

Diagram 2

Right Lobe of Liver
Inferior Vena Cava
Right Lower Lobe of Lung

Left Upper Lobe of Lung
Esophagus
Left Lower Lobe of Lung
Aorta

A

R   P   L

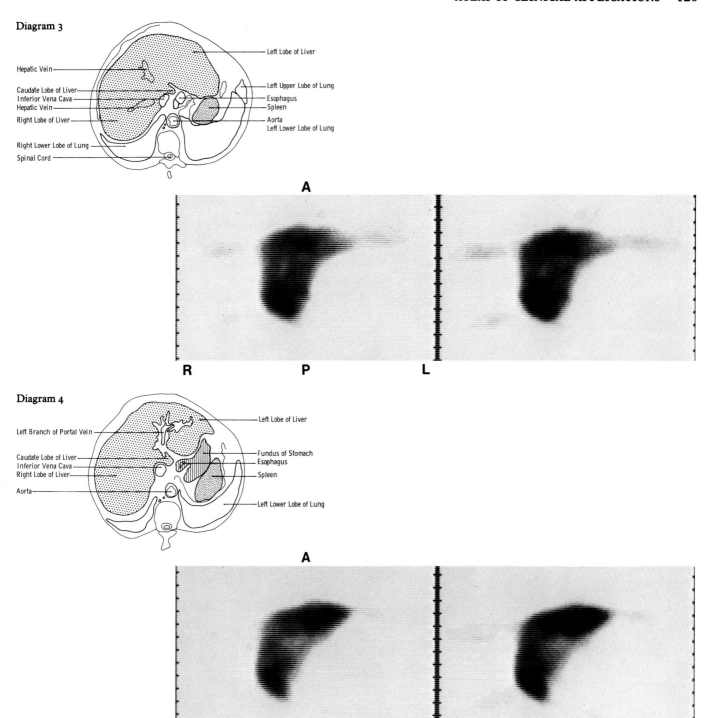

Diagram 3

Hepatic Vein

Caudate Lobe of Liver
Inferior Vena Cava
Hepatic Vein
Right Lobe of Liver

Right Lower Lobe of Lung
Spinal Cord

Left Lobe of Liver

Left Upper Lobe of Lung
Esophagus
Spleen
Aorta
Left Lower Lobe of Lung

A

R   P   L

Diagram 4

Left Branch of Portal Vein

Caudate Lobe of Liver
Inferior Vena Cava
Right Lobe of Liver

Aorta

Left Lobe of Liver

Fundus of Stomach
Esophagus
Spleen

Left Lower Lobe of Lung

A

R   P   L

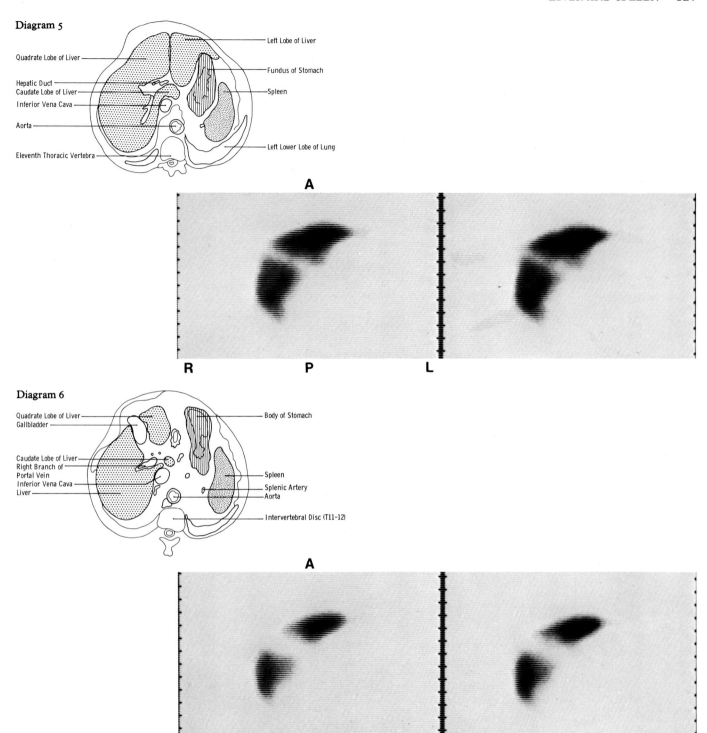

Diagram 5

Quadrate Lobe of Liver
Hepatic Duct
Caudate Lobe of Liver
Inferior Vena Cava
Aorta
Eleventh Thoracic Vertebra

Left Lobe of Liver
Fundus of Stomach
Spleen
Left Lower Lobe of Lung

A

R   P   L

Diagram 6

Quadrate Lobe of Liver
Gallbladder
Caudate Lobe of Liver
Right Branch of Portal Vein
Inferior Vena Cava
Liver

Body of Stomach
Spleen
Splenic Artery
Aorta
Intervertebral Disc (T11-12)

A

R   P   L

Diagram 7

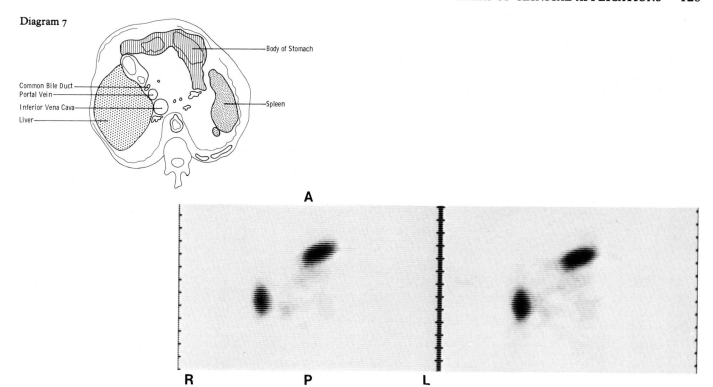

Patient 57

Diagnosis	50-year-old male with oat cell carcinoma of the bronchus. Referred for a liver scan.
Imaging	*Gamma camera scan.* Normal pattern of tracer distribution in the liver and spleen.
	CET scan. Note pattern of normal tomograms of the liver and spleen. Care must be exercised in the analysis of liver tomograms.

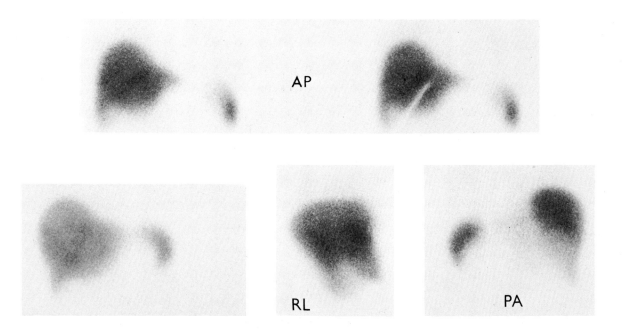

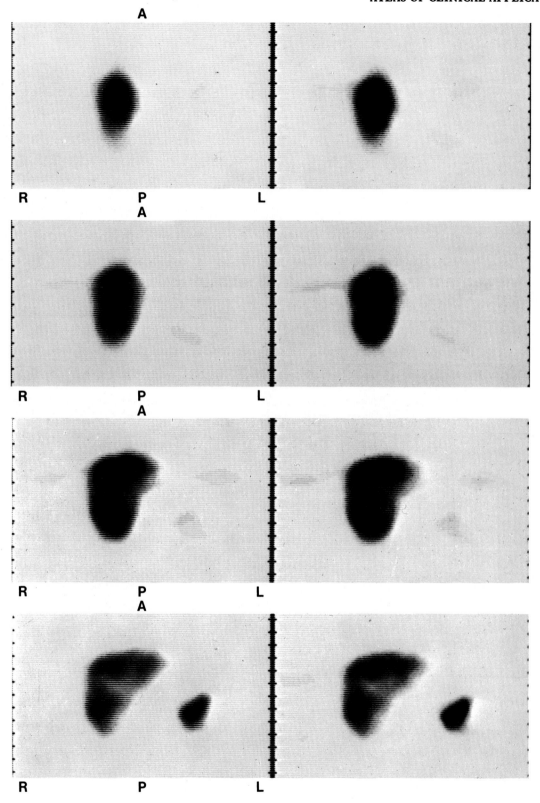

A

R P L

A

R P L

A

R P L

A

R P L

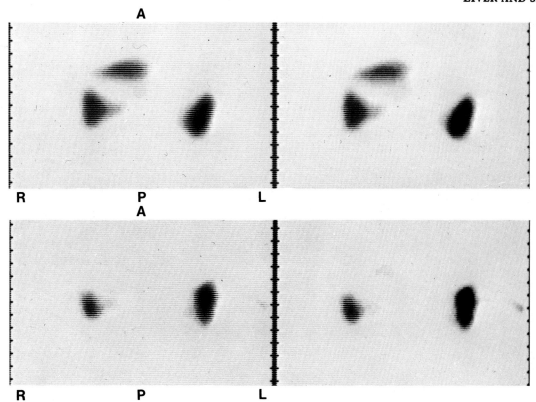

Patient 58

Diagnosis   Five-year-old child with Hodgkin's disease.

Imaging   *CET scan.* Note patchy uptake within enlarged liver and spleen.

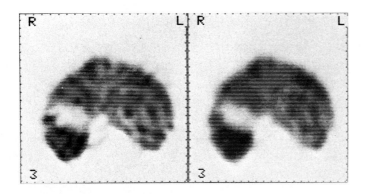 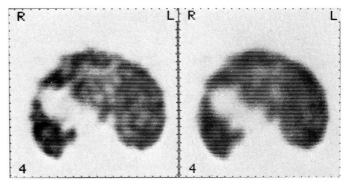

Patient 59

Diagnosis   40-year-old male with carcinoma of the stomach. Abnormal liver function tests. Jaundice.

Imaging   *CET scan.* Large, multiple, space occupying lesions in the liver. Normal tomograms of the spleen.

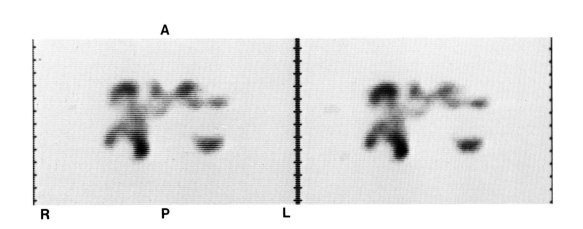

Patient 60

Diagnosis	40-year-old female patient with carcinoma of the breast. Raised alkaline phosphatase and raised ESR.
Imaging	*CET scan.* Multiple liver secondaries. Normal tomogram of the spleen.

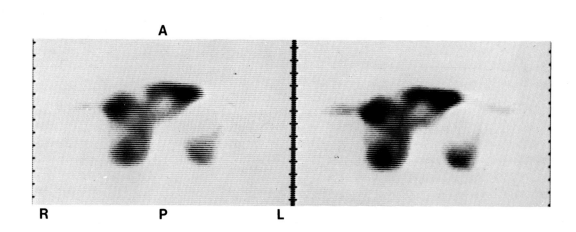

Patient 61

Clinical history   This 48-year-old female patient had a left mastectomy five years ago for carcinoma of the breast. Referred for routine screening.

Imaging   *Liver scan.* 5-view (erect and decubitus) gamma camera study. Patchy uptake of ^{99m}Tc sulphur colloid, particularly in the anterior projections.

CET scan. Tomograms show regular activity contours throughout the organ. No confirmatory evidence of space occupying disease in the liver. Normal tomograms of the spleen. Standard and magnified section scans shown. Normal ultrasound examination of the liver.

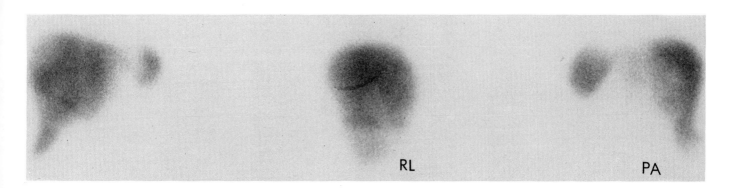

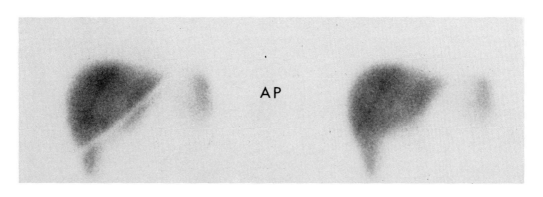

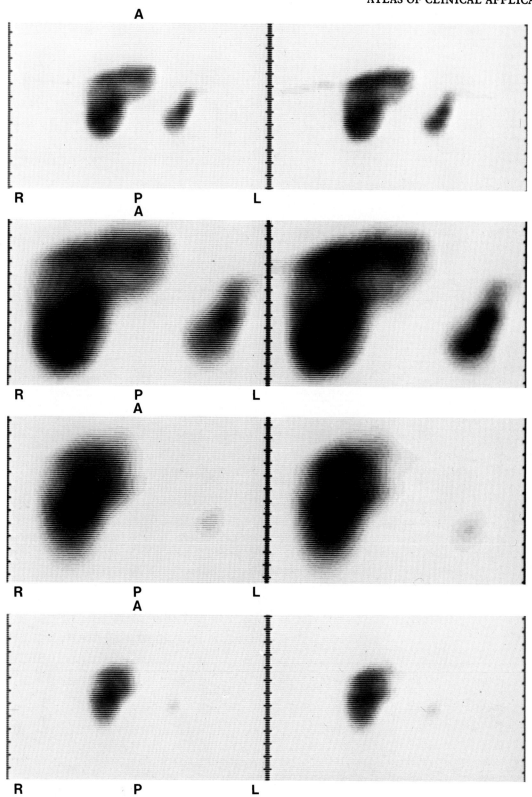

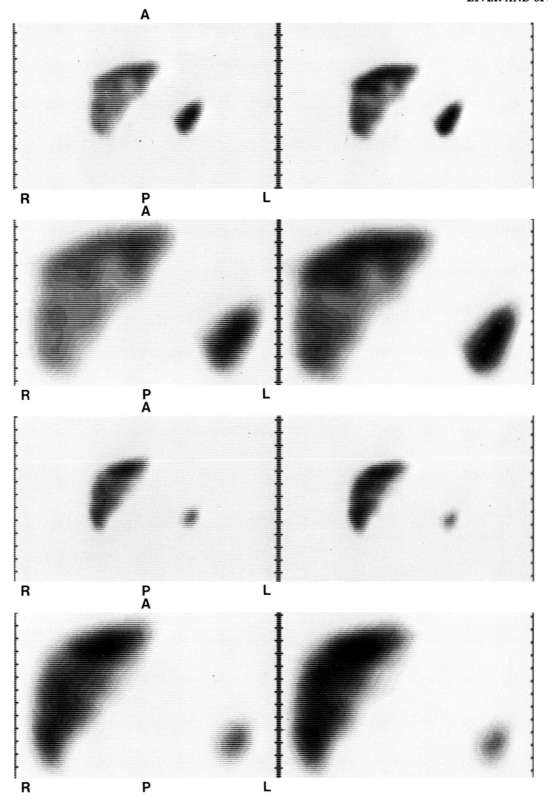

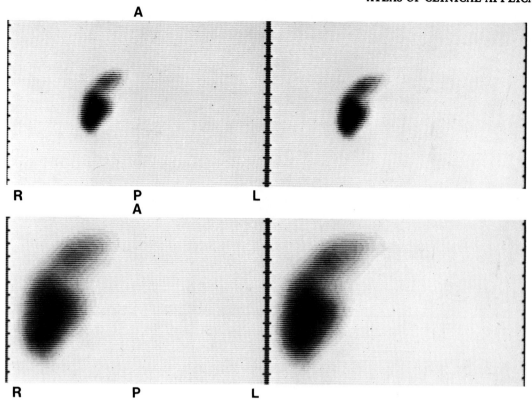

Patient 62

Clinical history This 50-year-old female patient had a carcinoma of the left breast removed two months previously. She was referred for routine screening.

Imaging *Liver scan.* Conventional liver scan shows a tracer uptake pattern which is suspicious, but not diagnostic of filling defects.

CET scan. Tomograms confirm irregular distribution of tracer with filling defects in the right lobe and in the interlobar region. Note injection artifact on tomogram 4. Normal tomograms of the spleen.
Ultrasound examination of the liver confirms the presence of liver secondaries.

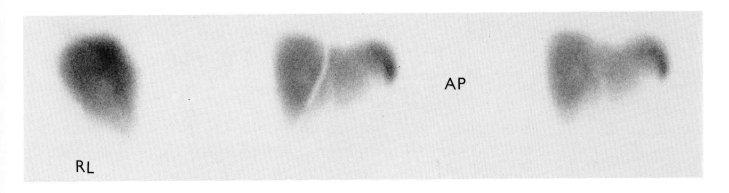

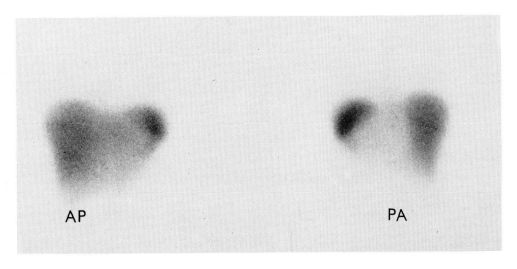

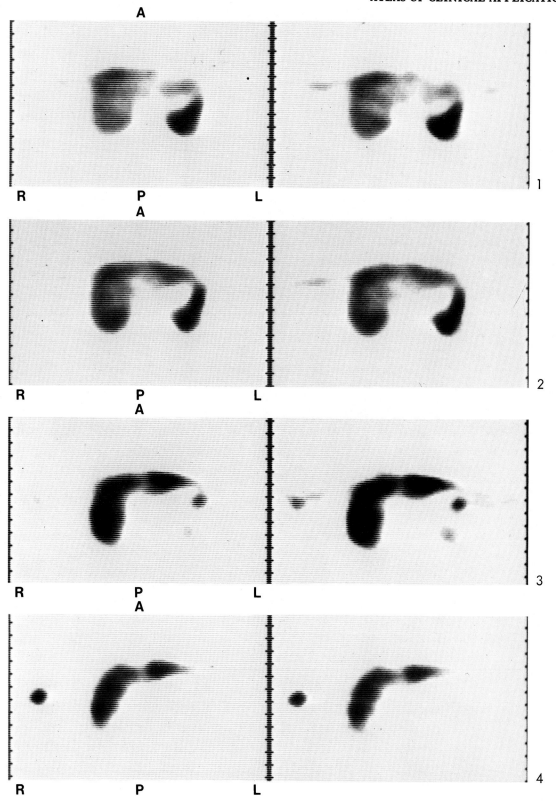

A

R   P   L
1

A

R   P   L
2

A

R   P   L
3

A

R   P   L
4

Patient 63

Diagnosis

44-year-old male patient with carcinoma of the larynx and right pleuritic pain.

Imaging

Liver scan. Gamma camera study reveals a large lesion within the right lobe of the liver.

CET scan. Tomograms confirm this lesion. *Liver secondaries.* Normal tomograms of the spleen.

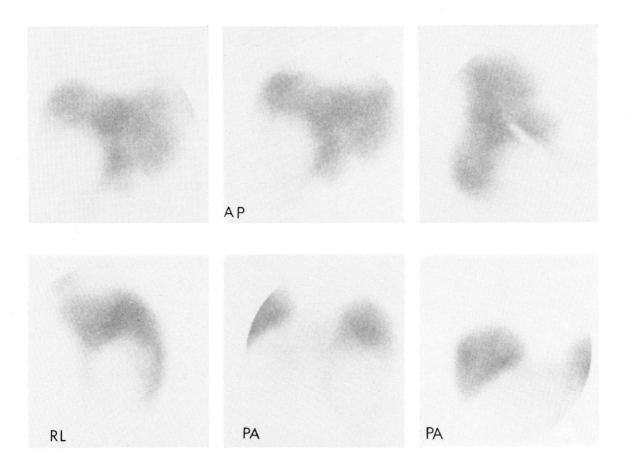

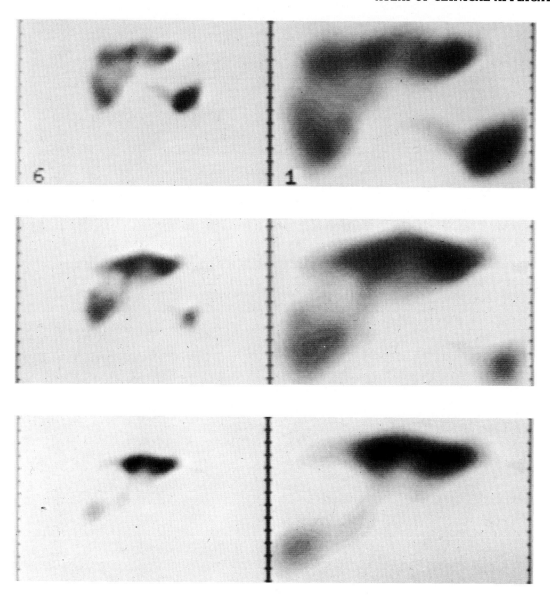

Patient 64

Clinical history   This 56-year-old female with adenosquamous carcinoma of the bladder presented with abdominal discomfort and abnormal liver function tests.

Imaging   *Gamma camera scan.* Evidence of a large filling defect in the middle of the right lobe (seen only in the posterior projection) and in the inferior aspect of the same lobe (seen in the anterior projections only).

CET scan. Tomograms confirm these lesions, well defined on sections one, two and three. Normal tomograms of a moderately enlarged spleen.

Outcome   Liver metastases.

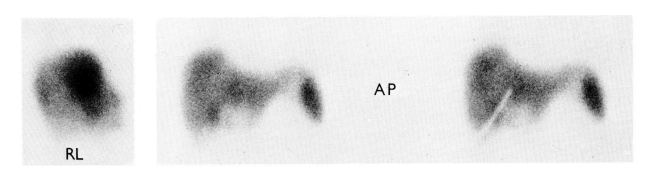

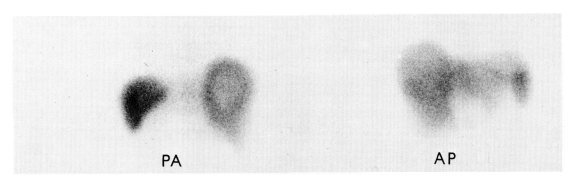

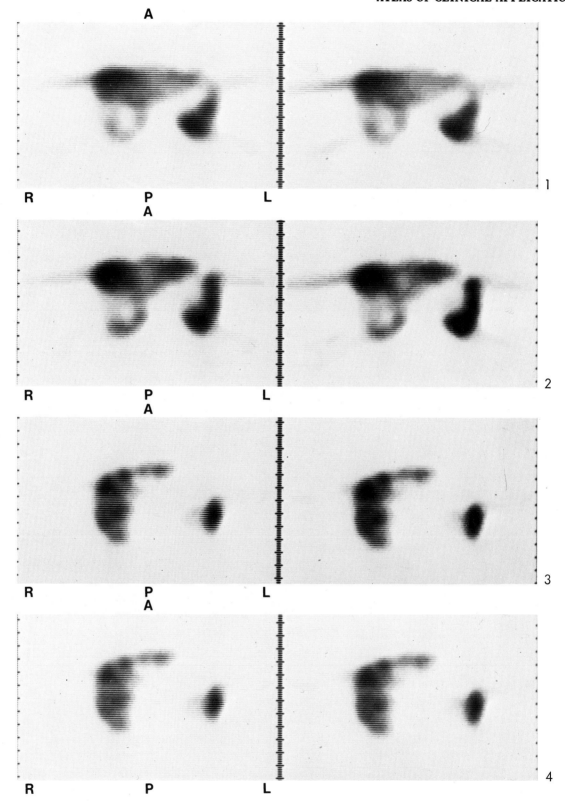

A

R   P   L

A

R   P   L

1

2

A

R   P   L

A

R   P   L

3

4

Patient 65

Clinical history

This 50-year-old male presented with chest pain and a mass seen on chest X-ray in the upper lobe of the left lung. He had moderate dyspnoea and pain in the right arm. Aspiration biopsy was negative, bronchoscopy failed. Referred for routine screening.

Imaging

Bone scan. Focal and abnormal uptake in the upper third of the right humerus.

Liver scan. Gamma camera study does not reveal focal involvement of the liver.

CET scan. Liver tomograms show regular distribution of tracer within the liver and spleen. No evidence of liver deposits.

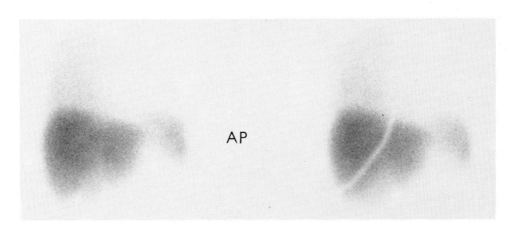

AP

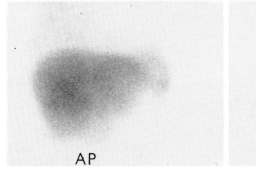

AP

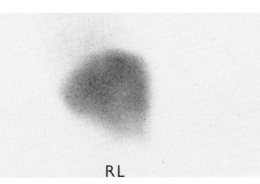

RL

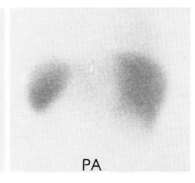

PA

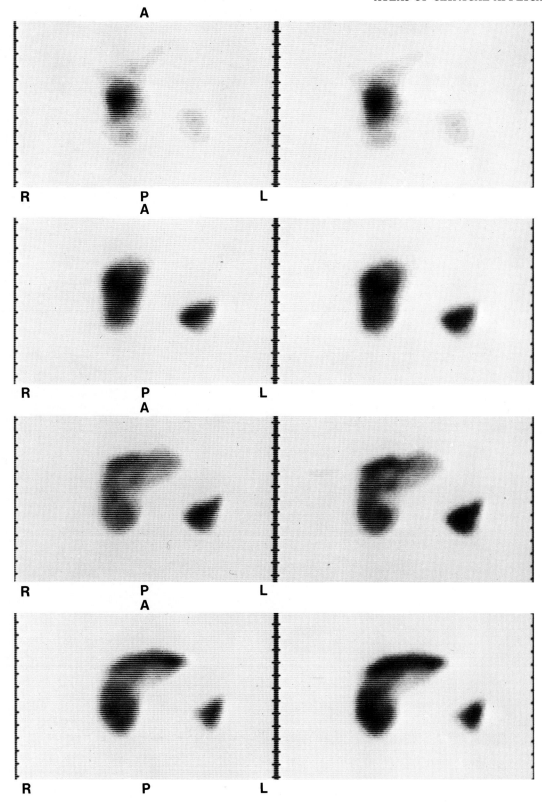

A

R   P   L

A

R   P   L

A

R   P   L

A

R   P   L

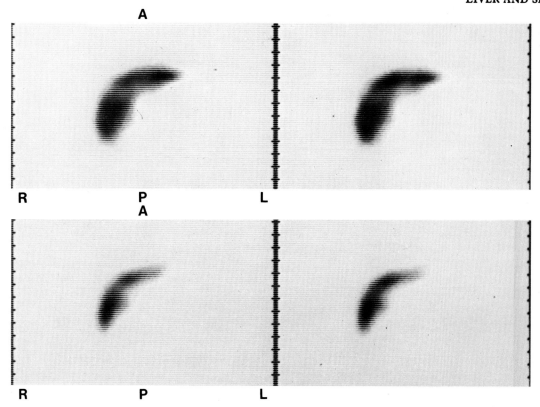

Patient 66

Clinical history   64-year-old man with known carcinoma of the bladder. Recent onset of paraesthesia and involuntary movements of the left arm and leg. Clinically, there was a suspicion of a right sided lesion, involving motor and sensory cortex.

Imaging   *CET brain scan.* A right sided parietal lesion is demonstrated. Perfusion sequence shows this lesion to be relatively avascular.

Liver scan. Gamma camera studies reveal hepatosplenomegaly and multiple filling defects in the liver compatable with liver secondaries.

CET liver scan. The liver tomograms reveal multiple well defined filling defects in both right and left lobes.

Outcome   Liver and brain secondaries from carcinoma of the bladder.

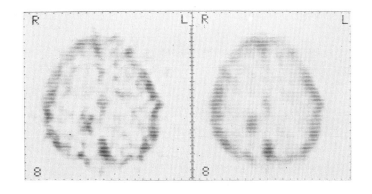

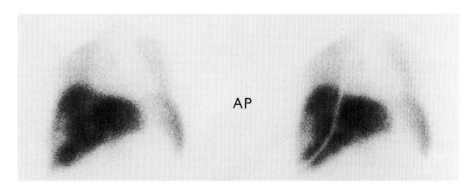

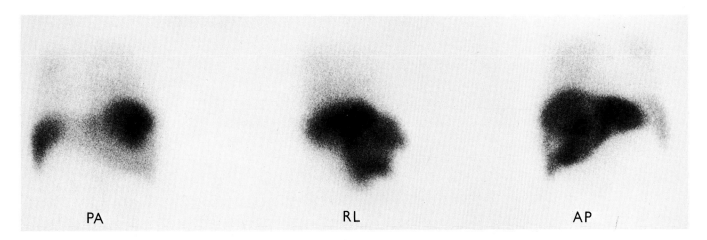

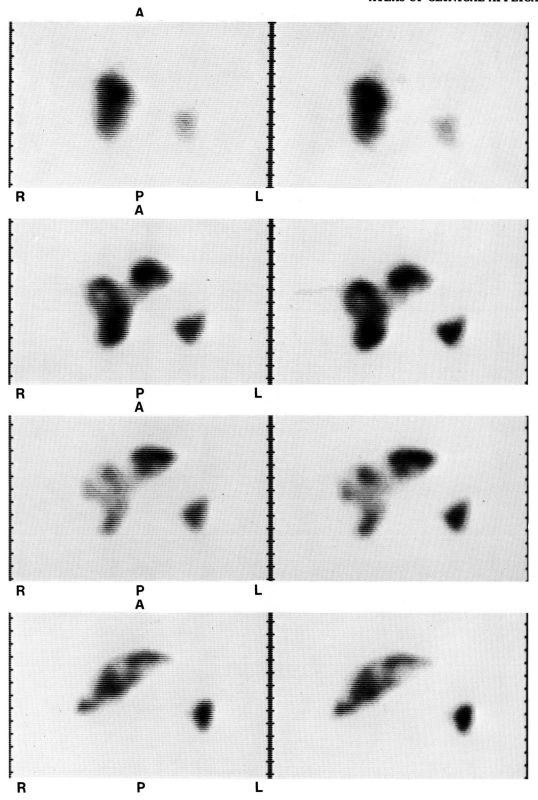

A

R   P   L

A

R   P   L

A

R   P   L

A

R   P   L

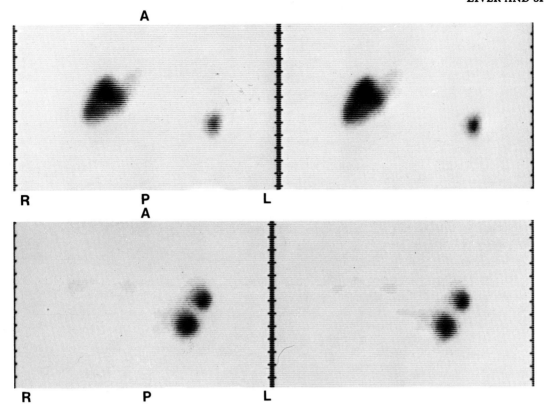

A

R   P   L

A

R   P   L

Patient 67

Clinical history   60-year-old male with carcinoma of the stomach. Post-gastrectomy. Cachexia.

Imaging   *Gamma camera scan.* Hepatomegaly. Multiple filling defects in the liver.

CET liver scan. Tomograms confirm the presence of multiple space occupying lesions.

Outcome   Liver metastases from carcinoma of the stomach.

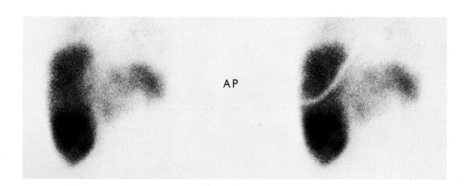

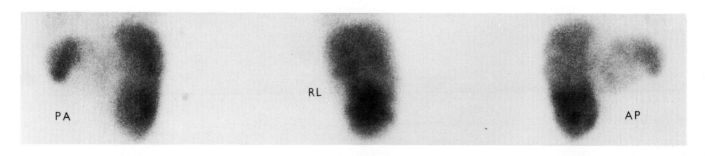

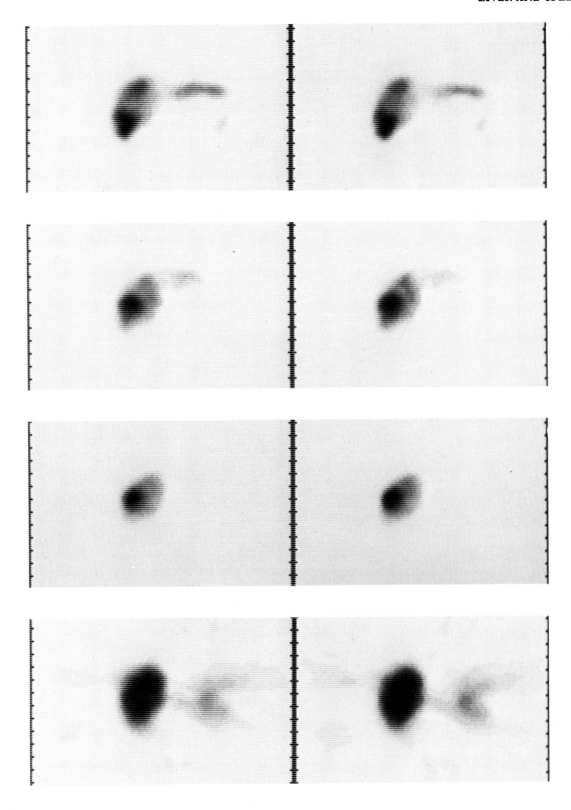

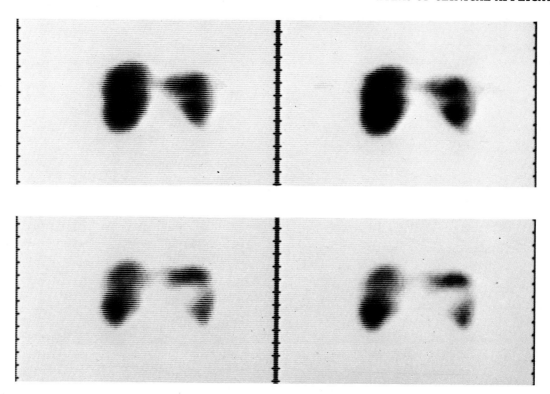

Patient 68

Diagnosis	61-year-old female with a lump in the left breast and axillary lymph nodes. Referred for routine screening.
Imaging	*Gamma camera liver scan.* Normal study.
	CET liver scan. Tomograms of liver and spleen confirm normal distribution of ^{99m}Tc sulphur colloid.

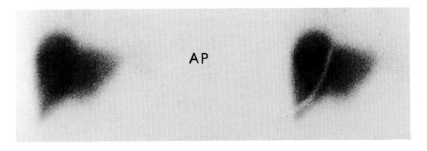

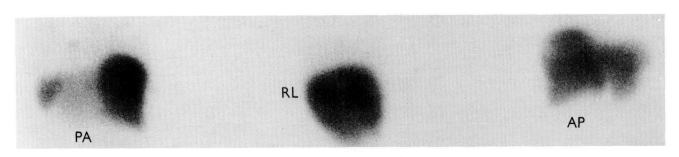

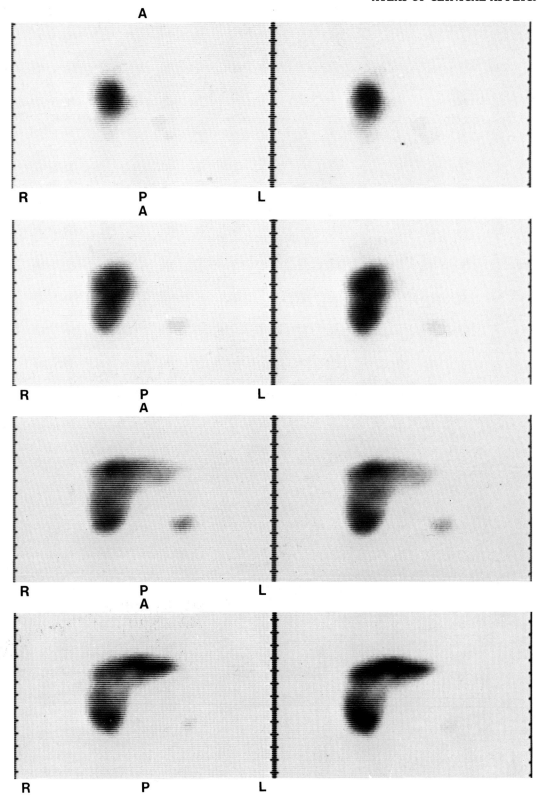

A

R   P   L

A

R   P   L

A

R   P   L

A

R   P   L

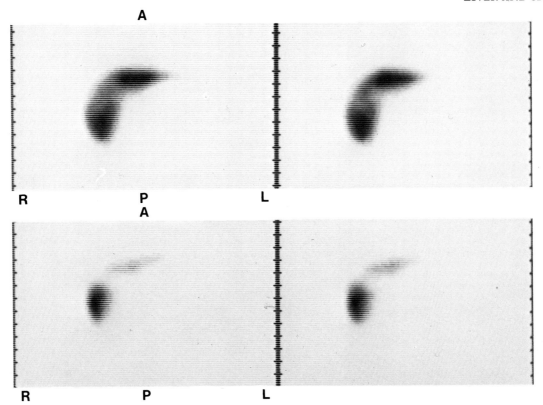

Patient 69

Clinical history

This 19-year-old man fell off a 9th floor balcony in Paris. There was an apparent single injury—fracture of the left wrist!

Ten days later, he developed severe abdominal pain, a mass was felt per rectum and a pelvic abscess was confirmed by ultrasound. There was no evidence of subphrenic collections, and on the ultrasound examination, liver and spleen were thought to be normal.

He had persistent pyrexia, raised white blood cell count and abnormal liver function tests.

Imaging

Gamma camera liver scan. There is a suggestion of small and multiple filling defects.

CET liver scan. Tomograms 4, 5 and 7 of the liver show clear evidence of filling defects within this organ, as a possible consequence of hepatic laceration. In addition, evidence of a subphrenic filling defect is obtained, best seen in tomograms 3 and 4.

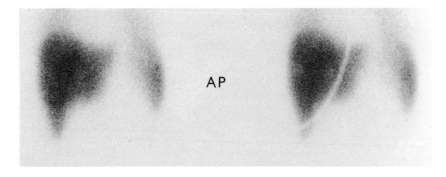

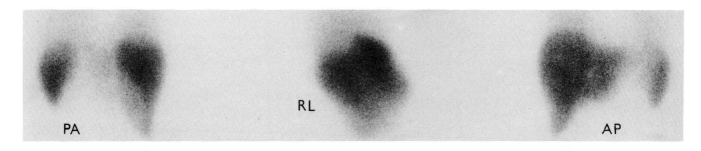

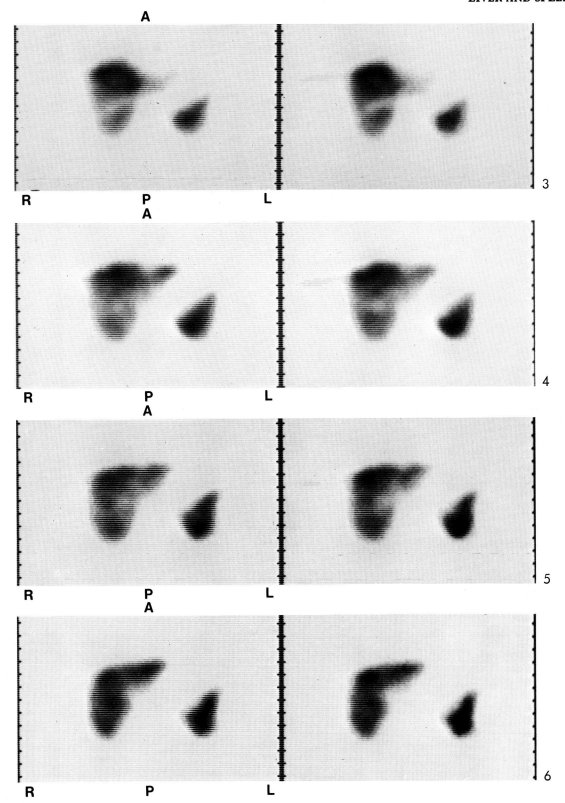

A

R   P   L

A

R   P   L

A

R   P   L

A

R   P   L

3

4

5

6

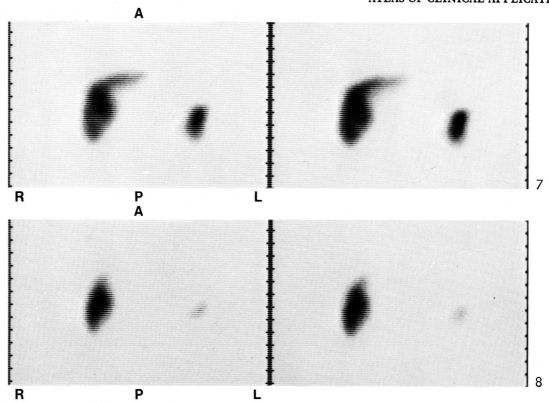

Patient 70

Clinical history   This female patient, aged 55, presented with carcinoma of the left breast six years ago. She represented with a local recurrence.

Imaging   *Liver scan.* Gamma camera studies reveal normal variations in liver anatomy with a pedunculate, mobile and prominent quadrate lobe of the liver. There is hepatomegaly but no evidence of focal disease. The apparent abnormalities of uptake in the lateral projections of the liver (RL) are due to the special configuration of the liver in this patient.

CET liver scan. The emission tomograms of the liver confirm the absence of disease; ultrasound examination also failed to show any evidence of space occupying disease of the liver.

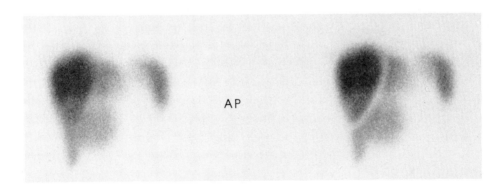

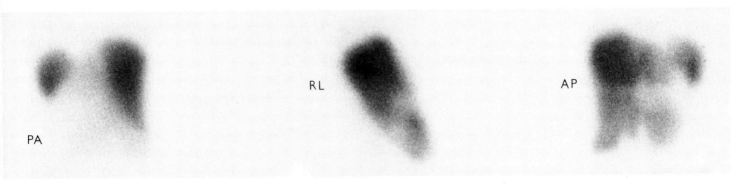

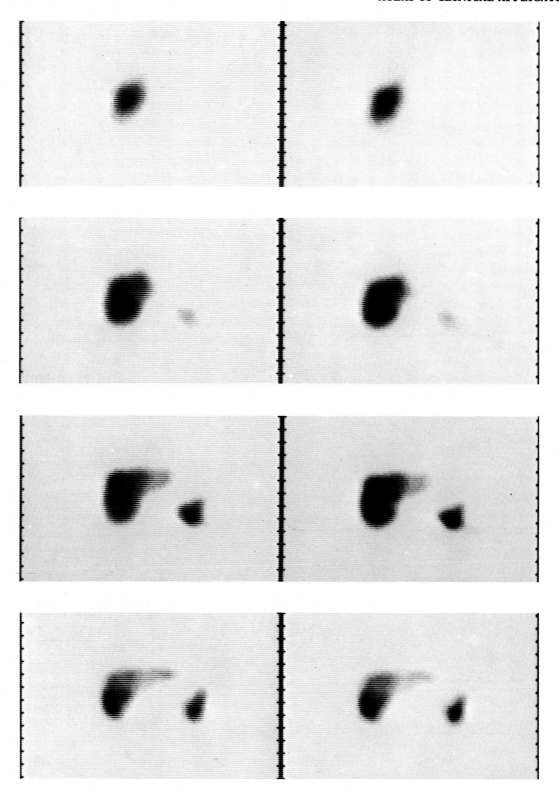

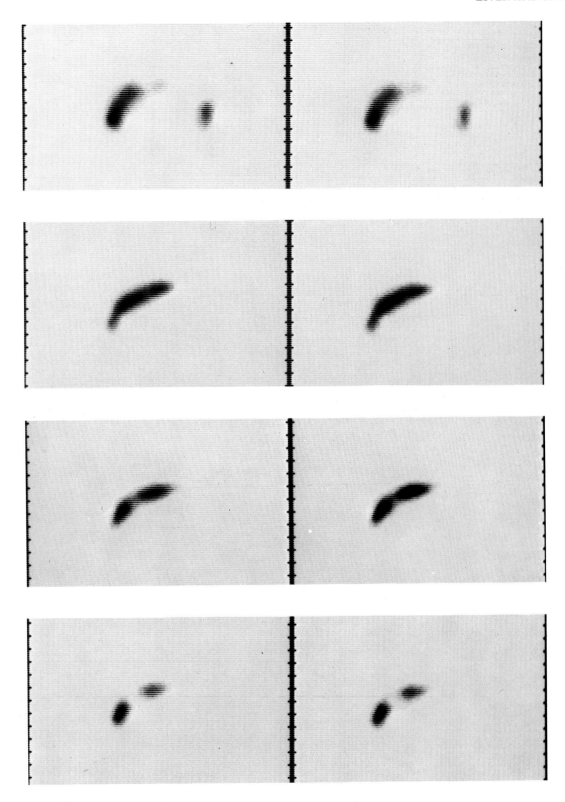

Patient 71

Clinical history

This 62-year-old female with known carcinoma of the right breast had a palpable liver and abnormal liver function tests. On ultrasound, there was a questionable large lesion in the left lobe of the liver. Referred for further investigation.

Imaging

Liver scan. Gamma camera studies confirm hepatomegaly. Pronounced porta hepatis. Large filling defect occupies majority of left lobe of liver.

CET liver scan. When a solitary and large lesion occupies the major part of an organ, tomographic techniques may be at a disadvantage. This is illustrated in this case, where the lesion is hidden; only with careful analysis of the liver tomograms, is the defect apparent—slice 4, arrow.

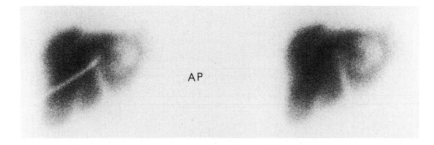

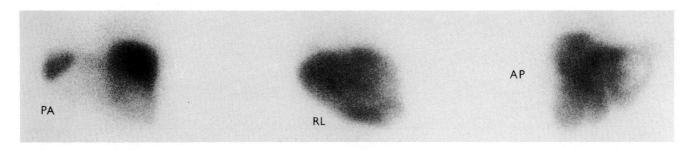

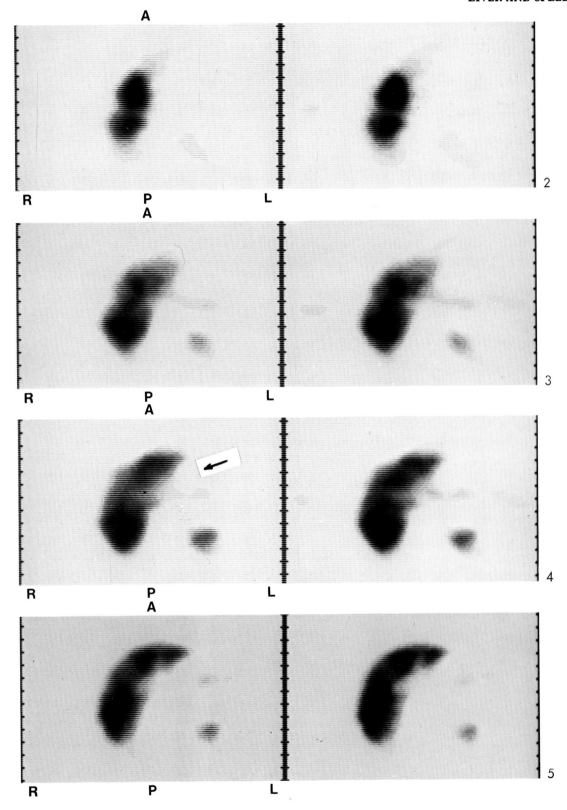

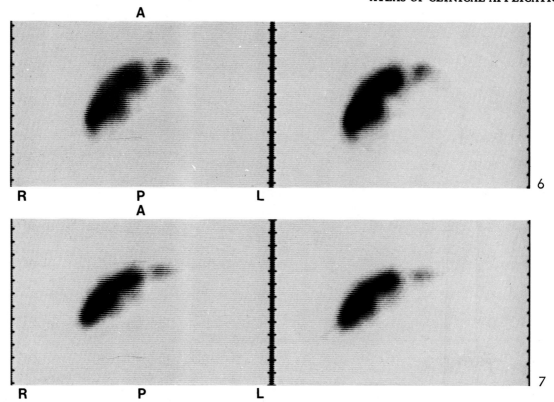

Heart

Patient 72

Diagnosis 42-year-old male with acute chest pain, borderline CK and ECG compatible with subendocardial necrosis.

Imaging *Gamma camera study.* Abnormal uptake (diffuse) over left precordium, suggestive of acute myocardial necrosis. Scan with ^{99m}Tc-IDP.

CET scan. Note considerable improvement in contrast resolution. Definite uptake within the left ventricle, diagnostic of acute myocardial necrosis.

Comment The benefit derived from improved contrast resolution may help in the diagnosis of the equivocal acute M.I. (small, posterior, subendocardial) and reduce the false negative rate.

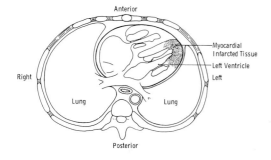

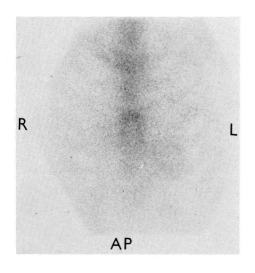

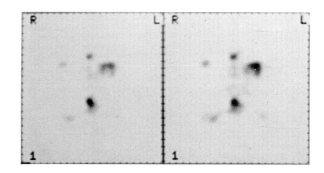

Patient 73

Diagnosis   Acute myocardial infarction, with positive ECG and raised enzymes.

Imaging   *CET scan.* Patient scanned with ^{99m}Tc-IDP 72 hours post infarction. Note tracer uptake in the necrosed left ventricle.

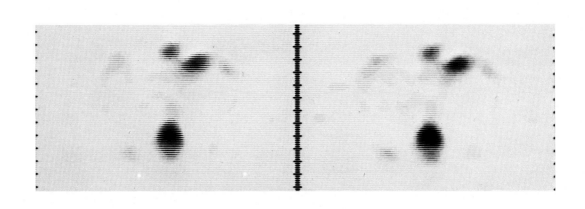

Patient 74

Diagnosis   Acute myocardial infarction.

Imaging   *CET scan.* Patient scanned with ^{99m}Tc-IDP 48 hours post infarction.
                         Demonstration of tracer uptake in damaged myocardium.

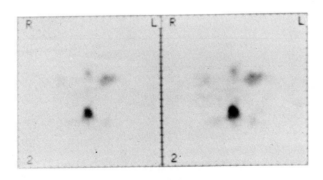

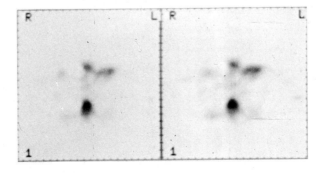

Patient 75

Diagnosis   Acute myocardial infarction.

Imaging   *CET scan.* Intense tracer (^{99m}Tc-IDP) uptake 48 hours after infarction.

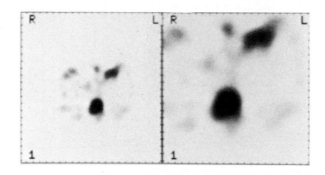

Lungs

Patient 76

Clinical history

This 63-year-old woman had a carcinoma of the cervix and was admitted for radiotherapy. There was a history of one week of breathlessness on slight exertion and a dull ache over lower right ribs, particularly when lying. No other signs or symptoms apart from palpitations.

Imaging

Gamma camera lung scan. Multiple projections reveal several areas of maintained ventilation but impaired perfusion typical of multiple pulmonary embolism.

CET scan. The severity of underperfusion of the left lung is well documented in these tomograms. In addition right upper lobe perfusion deficits are better visualized in these images than in the traditional 2 dimension Anger camera images.

DIAGRAMS A–F

NORMAL ANATOMY

Diagram A

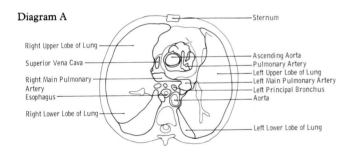

Diagram B

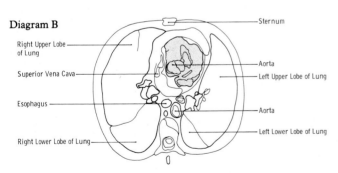

Diagram C

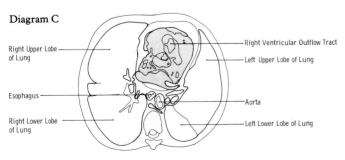

Diagram D

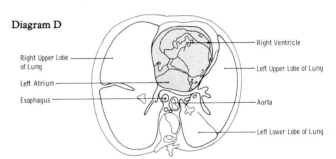

Diagram E

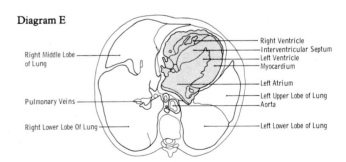

Diagram F

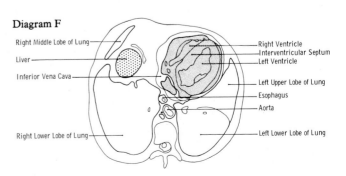

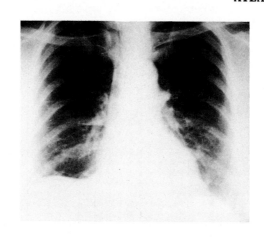

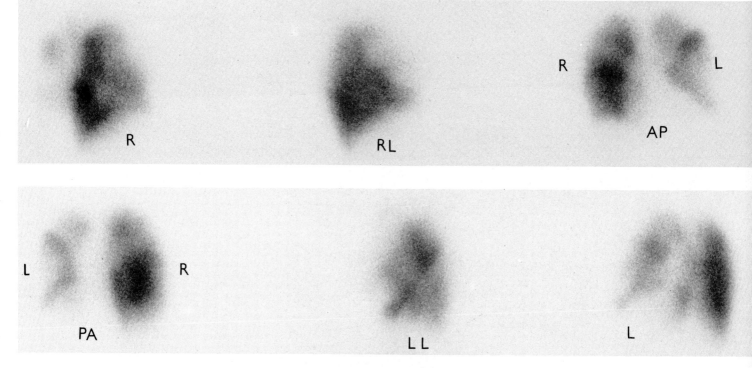

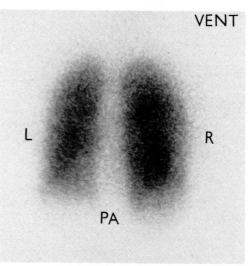

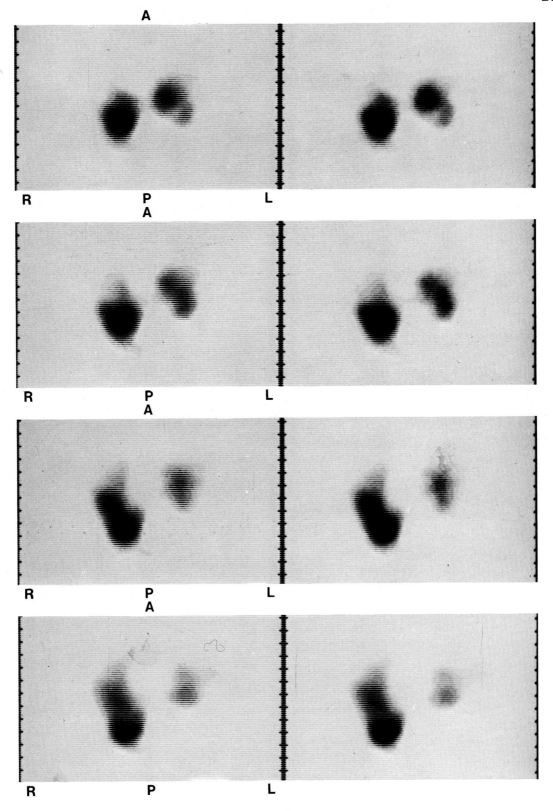

A

R P L

PA

R P L

PA

R P L

PA

R P L

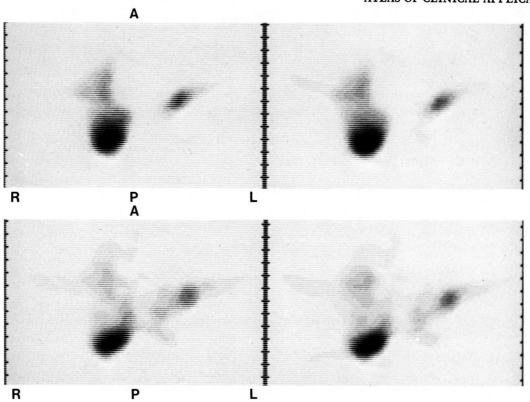

A

R   P   L

A

R   P   L

Patient 77

Clinical history

This 74-year-old male had a history of right sided heart failure and right pleural effusion—he suddenly developed symptoms and signs of a right sided deep vein thrombosis of the calf, chest pain and dyspnoea. ?Multiple pulmonary embolism.

Imaging

Lung scan. Gamma camera perfusion studies of the lung obtained with ^{99m}Tc albumin microspheres. Note symmetrical distribution of the radiopharmaceutical in all projections.

CET lung scan. Multiple emission tomograms of the lungs do not reveal focal perfusion deficit. Symmetrical perfusion patterns are observed. Note abnormal and enlarged mediastinal space.

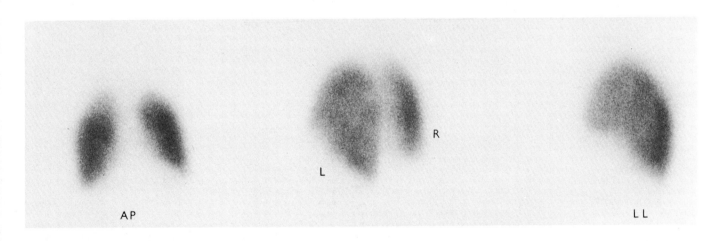

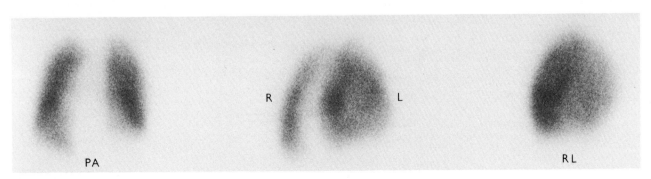

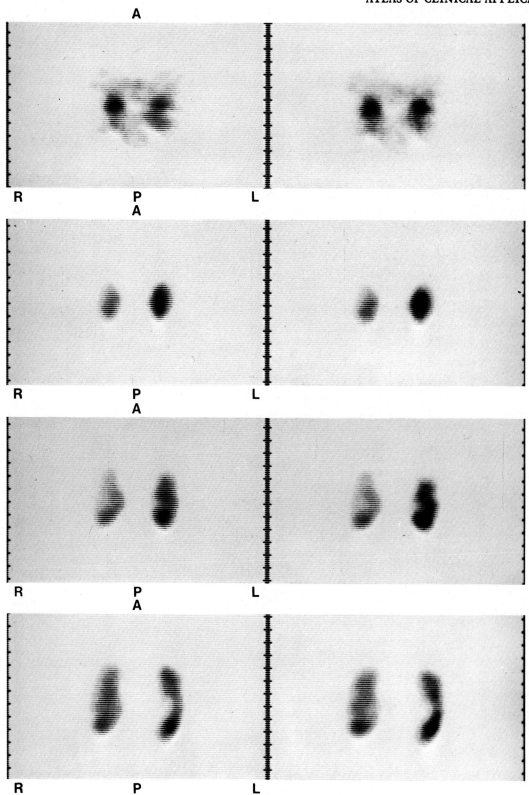

A

R   P   L

A

R   P   L

A

R   P   L

A

R   P   L

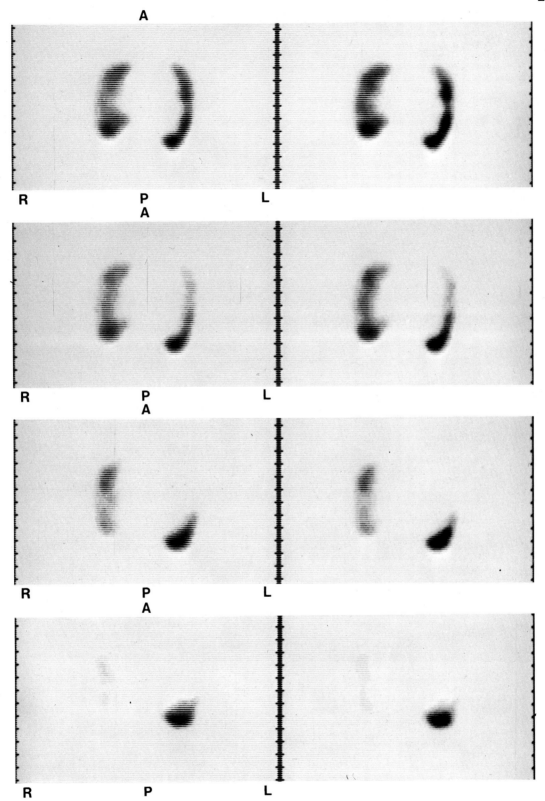

Patient 78

Diagnosis 55-year-old male with recurrent and multiple pulmonary embolism.

Imaging *Lung scan.* Gamma camera perfusion studies with ^{99m}Tc albumin microspheres confirm the presence of several areas of impaired perfusion in both lungs. These appear with a segmental distribution and are compatible with embolic disease.

CET lung scan. Emission tomograms of both lungs clearly show multiple perfusion defects. The total impairment of perfusion is better judged in these tomograms, with the right lung more impaired than the left. The maediastinal space is normal.

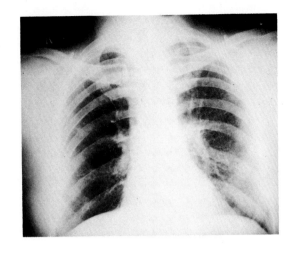

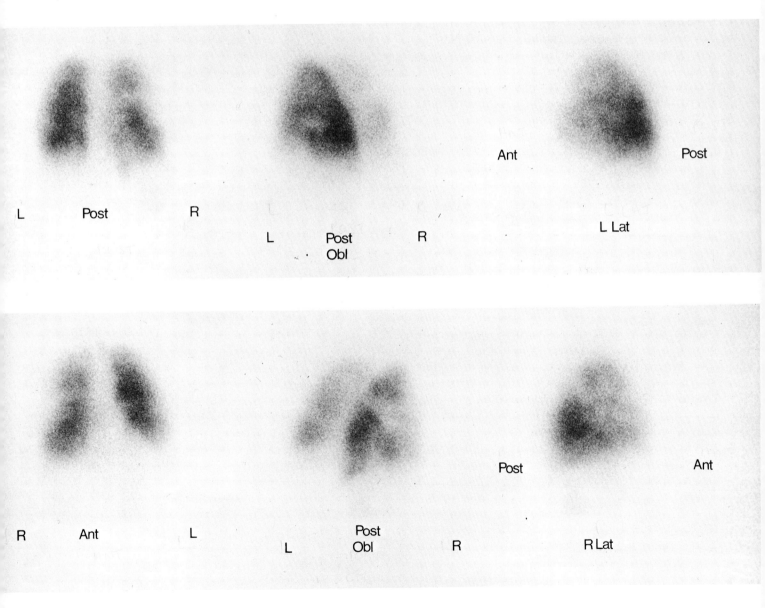

L   Post   R

L   Post   R
           Obl

Ant   Post

L Lat

R   Ant   L

L   Post   R
           Obl

Post   Ant

R Lat

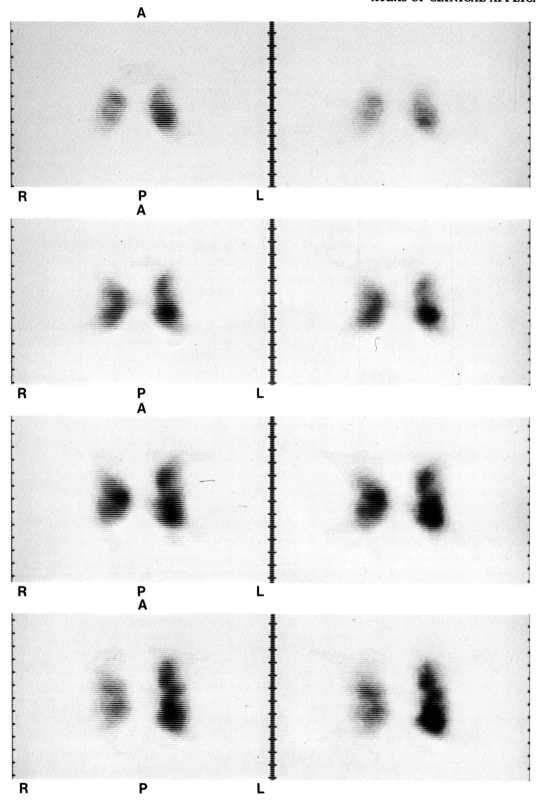

A

R   P   L
A

R   P   L
A

R   P   L
A

R   P   L

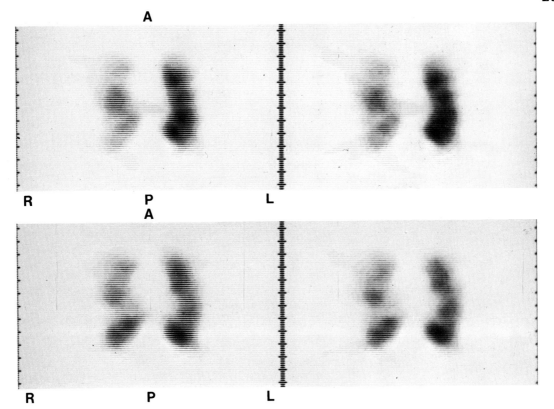

Patient 79

Clinical history   This 28-year-old female was on oral contraceptives for 5 years. She suffered from chest pain and dyspnoea 2 days before admission. An ECG pattern suggestive of pulmonary embolism was found.

Imaging   *Lung scan.* Gamma camera studies with ^{99m}Tc albumin microspheres. Multiple projections (including oblique views) fail to show clear segmental areas of hypoperfusion. The pattern is however not entirely normal.

CET lung scan. Multiple emission transaxial tomograms of the lungs do not show well defined (focal) areas of underperfusion. However the right lung is clearly underperfused, when compared to the left lung.

Outcome   The patient was anticoagulated and improved. A repeat CET lung scan showed marked improvement in the asymmetry of the perfusion to the right lung. Pulmonary embolism was thought to be the most likely cause!

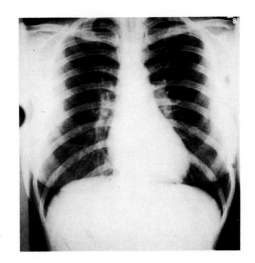

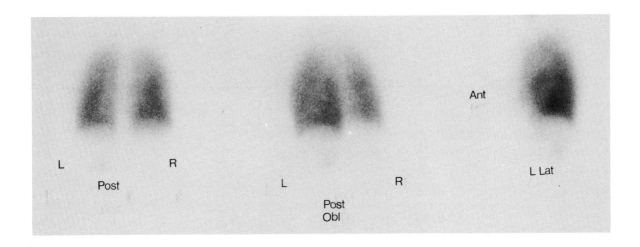

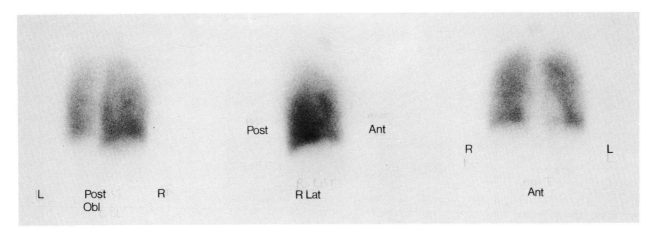

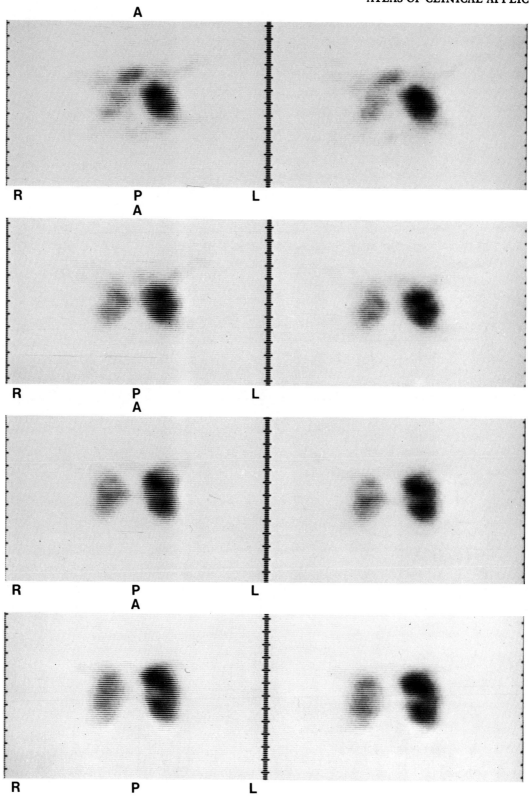

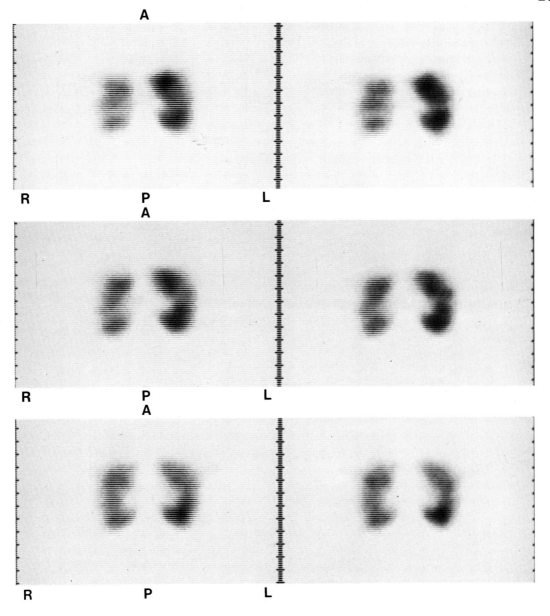

Patient 80

Clinical history

This 19-year-old female was on oral contraceptives. She had a two week history of pleuritic chest pain on the right side, below the shoulder blade. No other symptoms or signs.

Imaging

Lung scan. Gamma camera perfusion study with ^{99m}Tc albumin microspheres. Multiple projections. 2 perfusion defects seen—one at the base of the right lung (only moderately prominent)—and a second one at the base of the left lung.

CET lung scan. Emission tomography facilitates final interpretation. Sections 1–4 are entirely normal. Sections 5 and 6 reveal a clear perfusion deficit at the base of the right lung and confirm the normality of the perfusion of the base of the left lung. (On the gamma camera study, the heart is responsible for the pattern seen at the base.)

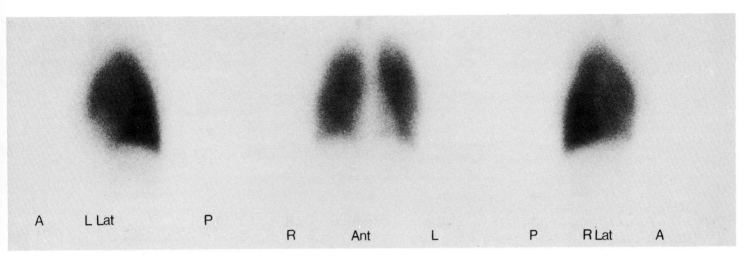

A L Lat P R Ant L P R Lat A

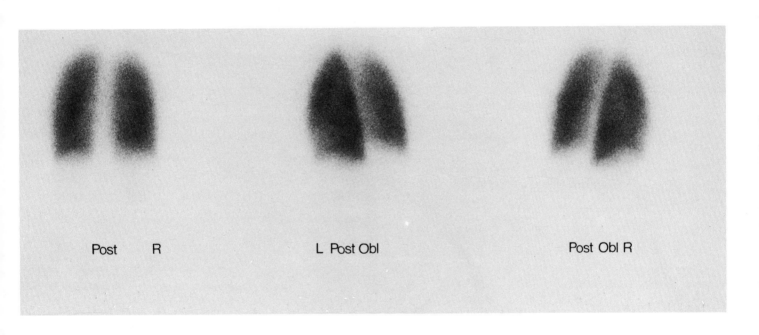

Post R L Post Obl Post Obl R

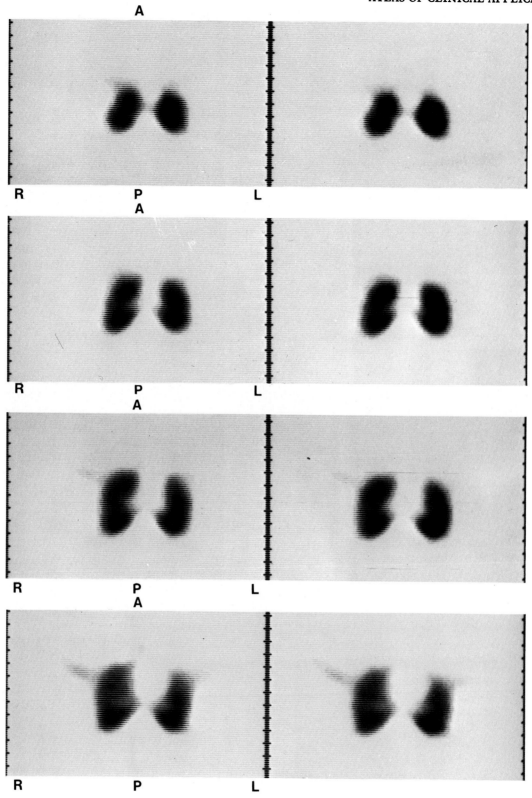

A

R　　　　P　　　　L
A

R　　　　P　　　　L
A

R　　　　P　　　　L
A

R　　　　P　　　　L

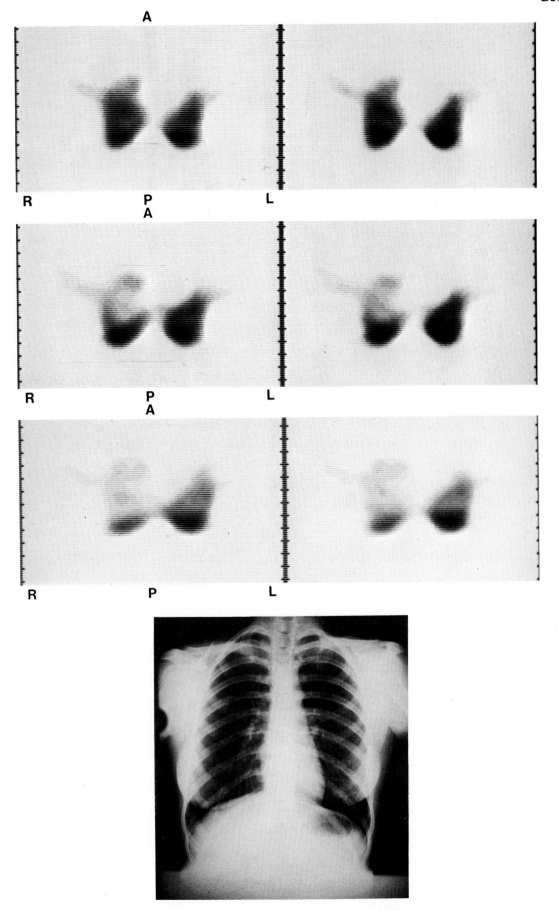

A

R P A L

R P A L

R P L

3. EMISSION AND TRANSMISSION BRAIN TOMOGRAPHY IN 208 PATIENTS

P. J. ELL AND J. M. DEACON
The Middlesex Hospital Medical School, London, U.K.

D. DUCASSOU AND A. BRENDEL
Hôpital du Haut Leveque, Bordeaux, France.

SUMMARY

Comparative emission (CET) and transmission (CTT) brain tomograms were obtained in 208 patients in order to establish the diagnostic accuracy of a new emission tomographic scanner in the detection of space occupying disease in the brain.

Concordant results were obtained in 169 patients (81.25 per cent). CTT scanning led to an overall false positive rate of 0.48 per cent and a false negative rate of 6.25 per cent. CET scanning led to a false positive rate of 0 per cent and a false negative rate for malignant disease of 2.40 per cent and for vascular disease of 10.10 per cent. The higher CET false negative rate for vascular disease is related to the CTT detection of old infarction. For recent vascular disease, CET and CTT detection rate is identical.

CET imaging is shown to be highly sensitive in the detection of space occupying pathology in the brain. It represents an ideal screening procedure.

INTRODUCTION

There is renewed interest in the clinical potential of computerized emission tomography (Kan & Hopkins 1979, Vogel et al 1978, Ell et al 1979). Significant improvement in the technical solutions offered by specialized instrumentation for the recording of emission tomograms and initial clinical results were published by us last year (Ell et al 1978). Since then, we have aimed at the establishment of the place and clinical value of CET scanning in the screening and detection of intracranial space occupying disease when confronted with now conventional CTT imaging. A trial was organized between the two European centres involved in the evaluation of a new emission tomographic brain scanner (Jarritt et al 1979). Since March 1978, data on 208 patients with emission and transmission brain tomograms were collected in London and Bordeaux.

PATIENTS AND METHODS

208 patients referred for the investigation of space occupying pathology in the brain were investigated. All had full clinical examination, emission and transmission brain tomograms and whenever relevant EEG's and/or angiograms. All patients had radionuclide angiography carried out and 75 per cent of them had also conventional 4-view Anger gamma camera studies.

Emission tomography was carried out on the Cleon-710 tomographic brain imager. A standard dose of ^{99m}Technetium-pertechnetate was given intravenously (15–20 mCi) and tomographic scanning commenced one hour post injection. The scanner was operated with window settings for ^{99m}Technetium (130–170 KeV), a scan time of four minutes per slice and slice spacing of 1.25 cm. A fixed background cut-off of 25 per cent was chosen.

Transmission tomography was carried out in London on the EMI CT5005 scanner, a scan time of 20 seconds per slice and slice spacing between 8–13 mm. All patients had studies performed with and without contrast material. In Bordeaux, the transmission tomograms of the brain, again with and without contrast, were recorded on a CGR ND 8000 scanner, with a scan time of 40 seconds per slice and slice spacing of 5 mm.

Reporting of data was done independently in London and Bordeaux. In both centres, CET and CTT scans were also reported independently.

The clinical material falls into three categories: malignant disease (which comprises primary or secondary tumours of the brain), vascular disease (which comprises cerebrovascular accidents, haematomata, subdural haematomata and arteriovenous malformation) and normals (patients where clinical history and outcome and silent transmission and emission tomograms failed to show evidence for intracranial space occupying disease).

RESULTS

Group A

Concordant CET and CTT data were obtained in 169 patients (81.25 per cent). There were 74 patients with malignant disease, 58 patients with vascular disease and 37 patients were judged as normal.

Discordant CET and CTT data were obtained in 39 patients.

Group B

In 13 cases (6.25 per cent) the CTT scan was negative in the presence of a positive CET scan. Of these 13 cases, three were caused by malignant disease and 10 cases were caused by vascular disease.

Group C

In 26 cases (12.50 per cent) the CET scan was negative in the presence of a positive CTT scan. Of these 26 cases, five were caused by malignant disease and 21 cases were caused by vascular disease.

CET imaging had a false positive rate of 0 per cent. CTT imaging had a false positive rate of 0.48 per cent.

CET imaging had a false negative rate of 2.40 per cent (malignant disease) and 10.10 per cent (vascular disease). CTT imaging had a false negative rate of 1.44 per cent (malignant disease) and of 4.80 per cent (vascular disease).

DISCUSSION

Group A

There was a high percentage of concordant CET and CTT results. From the 74 patients with malignant disease, 26 had multiple cerebral secondaries from a variety of primary tumours, the remaining 48 patients had primary brain neoplasms. From the 58 patients with vascular disease, there were nine intracerebral haematomata, two chronic subdural haematomata, one arteriovenous malformation and 46 infarcts.

Group B

From the 13 cases with a false negative CTT scan, there was one patient with a parietal glioma, two patients with multiple cerebral secondaries, two patients with isodense chronic subdural haematomata and eight patients with infarcts.

Group C

From the five malignant cases with a false negative CET scan, there was one patient with multiple cerebral metastases, one astrocytoma, one frontal and one parietal glioma and one case shown at operation to be due to an epidermoid cyst.

From the 21 vascular cases with a false negative CET scan, there was one patient with bilateral chronic subdural haematomata, 11 cases with more than seven week old infarcts and nine cases less than five days old.

It is clear from this data that CET scanning is highly sensitive in the detection of intracranial space occupying disease. It represents a significant improvement over conventional Anger gamma camera imaging. Indeed, 5 per cent of all lesions were detected only on the CET scanner when compared with the detectability achieved with the gamma cameras. However, in approximately 20 per cent of all cases, lesion localization in depth was significantly improved by CET scanning. This was particularly apparent in the differential diagnosis of skull from brain secondaries, in the precise localization of lesions in the cerebellopontine angle, posterior fossa and base of the brain. Only 75 per cent of all cases were scanned simultaneously with Anger gamma cameras, since one of the two centres involved in this study no longer considered gamma camera studies justified due to the superior imaging characteristics of the emission tomographic scanner.

It is also apparent from this study that a high CET false negative rate for vascular disease was recorded. However, this mainly occurs as a consequence of the known CTT detection of old infarction. In very early cerebrovascular disease (less than five days), CET scanning will also be negative due to absent tracer concentration in the lesion. In terms of detection (sensitivity) this remains a drawback for CET scanning. If these patients are scanned during the two week period where tracer concentration peaks within the lesion, CET and CTT scanning achieve the same pick-up rate—this explains the high percentage of concordant results obtained in the patients with vascular disease in group A. In addition, it is worthwhile to note that CTT scanning has a small but real false negative rate in isodense vascular disease, as shown in group B.

In this series, CET scanning had a remarkable 0 per cent false positive rate and a very low false negative rate (2.40 per cent) in the detection of primary or secondary intracranial neoplasms.

Emission tomography is becoming more available. Within the last year, seven centres (at least) emerged in the U.K. alone with the technical infrastructure required to record computerized emission tomograms. We do not doubt that further work will progressively demonstrate its clinical potential.

REFERENCES

Ell P J, Jarritt P H, Deacon J M, Brown N J G 1978 Lancet II: 608–610
Ell P J, Jarritt P H, Langford R, Pearce P C, Deacon J M 1979 Fortsch. Roentgenst. und Nuklearmedizin 4: 499–507
Jarritt P H, Ell P J, Myers M J, Brown N J G, Deacon J M 1979 Journal of Nuclear Medicine 20: 319–328
Kan M K, Hopkins G B 1979 Journal of Nuclear Medicine 20: 514–521
Vogel R A, Kirch D, LeFree M, Steele P 1978 Journal of Nuclear Medicine 19: 648–654

4. THE CLEON-710 TOMOGRAPHIC BRAIN IMAGER

The Cleon-710 imager uses a number of moving radiation detectors with short focal length collimators, having a wide angle of acceptance for emitted photons. These are mounted in the gantry assembly (Fig. 4.1). Operator interaction is via the console and hand held control for manual couch operation. The principles of operation of this device will be considered in this chapter together with its physical performance characteristics.

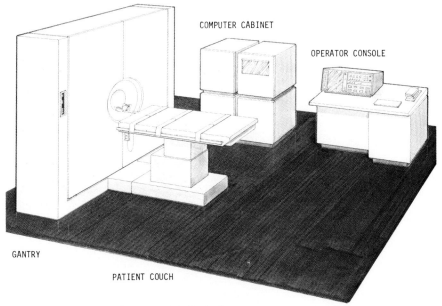

Fig. 4.1   The Cleon-710 Tomographic Brain Imager.

PRINCIPLES OF OPERATION

The gantry assembly contains 12 scanning detectors which are mounted on radial slide rails arranged in a clockwise fashion at 30° intervals around the opening, which has a diameter of 28.5 cm. Each detector consists of a focussing collimator (focal length 15 cm), a 20 × 13 × 2.5 cm NaI crystal, light guide, photomultiplier tube (9 cm diameter), amplifier and pulse height analyser (Fig. 4.2).

A focussing collimator consists of a number of tapered holes whose axes join at the so-called focal point. The distance of this point from the detector is referred to as the focal length. In the focal plane the visual field is small although there is a considerable region from within which gamma-ray photons may directly reach the crystal face and be detected. In the focal plane there is a rapid

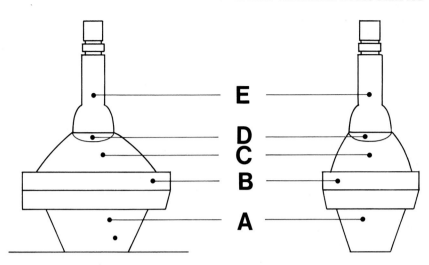

Fig. 4.2 Front and side view of detector assembly.
(A) Multichannel focused lead collimator.
(B) NaI(Tl) scintillation crystal.
(C) Polished light guide.
(D) Photocathode collection lens.
(E) Photomultiplier Tube.

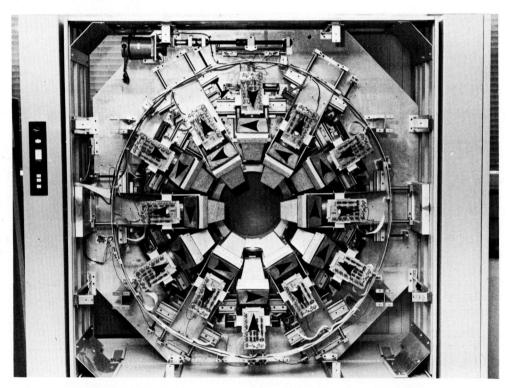

Fig. 4.3 Gantry detector assembly. Detectors positioned at mid-point of first scan line. The current motion is indicated together with their respective vertical step directions.

fall-off of sensitivity as a point source moves away from the focus. On the axis of the collimator other planes have lower sensitivities which usually vary less rapidly. The characteristics of such collimators are usually determined by measuring the response when the collimator scans across a radioactive line source. This shows the variation of sensitivity with distance at right angles to the axis. A commonly used index of resolution is the full width at half maximum of the curve (FWHM). (See *Radioisotopes in Medical Diagnosis*, ed. Belcher &

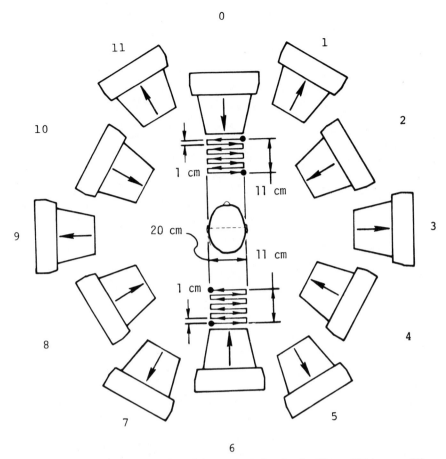

Fig. 4.4 Diagrammatic representation of detector motion for the Cleon-710 imager. The rectilinear motion causes the focal point of the detectors to scan half the field of view from different angles.

Vetter, Ch. 6.) FWHM values for the detector assembly are approximately 0.6 cm in the slice and 1.3 cm perpendicular to the slice, with a focal depth of 2.5 cm for energies below 300 keV. Note that these are the intrinsic characteristics of the detector assembly and not those of the reconstructed images. The limit of 300 keV is due both to collimator design and the limited amount of shielding surrounding the detector assembly. To make the enclosure as compact as possible, the detectors are offset physically and are mechanically coupled so that they do not all move in the same direction at the same time.

Figure 4.3 shows the detector positions during the initial scan line. The offset of the detectors is clearly seen (arrows indicating the initial motion of each detector have been inserted). The motion of the detectors is better illustrated in Figure 4.4. They move in pairs, in such a way that when one pair of detectors is scanning tangentially and is incremented towards the opening at the end of each line the adjacent pairs are scanning tangentially and are incremented away from the opening at the end of each line. The focal point of each detector scans half the region imaged. The focal point of each detector performs a rectilinear scan within the plane of the slice over the brain from a different angle, each detector performing 12 tangential line scans. At the end of each line each detector is incremented 1 cm towards or away from the centre. Each line scan is 20 cm long (the effective diameter of the region imaged) and is divided into 128 resolution elements. The resolution element associated with each element of these arrays measures 1.56 mm × 1 cm.

During the scanning process the output from each detector is sampled in rotation every 4.8 μsec. The output indicates whether valid photons have been detected during the preceding 4.8 μsec. (If more than a single valid event has occurred it will only be registered as a single event.) This gives a maximum linear counting rate of 200 000 cts/sec/detector. The data from the twelve detectors is multiplexed and transferred via the gantry data line to accumulators where the sampling and accumulation process continues until a resolution element has been traversed. The data in the accumulators is then transferred via a direct memory access (DMA) link into the computer memory where it is stored until a complete slice has been scanned. The spacing between slices can be selected in multiples of 3 mm and is automatically controlled by the patient couch movement. (The number of slices to be sequentially scanned is selected on the console prior to the study.) To aid in positioning the patient and the acquisition of appropriate slices the gantry can be tilted through an angle of $\pm 20°$ to the vertical. It should be noted that the slice spacing requested refers to couch motion perpendicular to the slice at zero gantry rotation. A correction is automatically applied to this value to maintain the required spacing in these inclined planes.

GANTRY CALIBRATION

Tomographic techniques require that the centre of rotation of the instrument be strictly controlled in order to avoid reconstruction artefacts. The initial calibration of the Cleon-710 requires the calculation of two offset values for each detector which correct for error in the position of the focal point relative to the centre of the field to view when the detector is positioned at the mechanical centre of the innermost scan line. Corrections for variations in detector geometry perpendicular to the slice are not applied and result in an increase in slice thickness and a reduction in sensitivity compared with the theoretical values. The lateral shifts and variable focal depth positions arise from two sources. (a) The inaccuracies in the mechanical alignment of the system. (b) The variability in the collimator casting. The magnitude of these errors although small is significant and they are corrected for as follows:

The vertical offsets are derived from the measured collimator characteristics. The horizontal offsets are calculated by scanning a point source at the centre of the field and then minimizing the difference between raster scans obtained from opposing detector pairs. The time interval required between recalibrations is dependent on the mechanical stability of the instrument and is typically several months. A daily routine check on this calibration is provided by a ring phantom which should reconstruct as a circle (Fig. 4.5). This is also used to adjust the energy setting of the individual detectors using the facility provided which allows all the detectors to be positioned equidistant from the source. By careful matching of collimator and photomultiplier assemblies, approximately equal sensitivities are obtained for each of the detectors over the range of energies used. Small variations in sensitivity are corrected for during the reconstruction process as follows: opposing detector pairs scan the central portion of the field from the same angle and the superimposed central scan line data are used to normalize the response of opposing pairs of detectors. The raw count sums for the six pairs of detectors are then normalized to each other yielding twelve normalization factors.

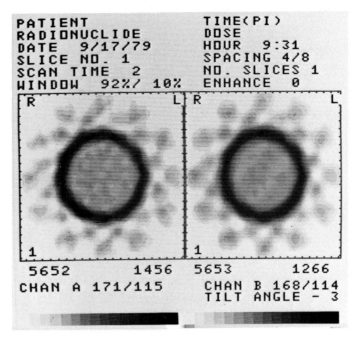

Fig. 4.5   Ring phantom calibration image.

DATA PROCESSING

Data processing is performed using a Data General S/230 Eclipse computer with 48K of memory. This is interfaced to dual floppy diskette drives for patient data storage, and to a disk drive unit for a dual platter hard disk, giving intermediate data and program storage.

The data input consists of 12 rectilinear scans each 128×12 elements. This data is shifted by the horizontal and vertical offset values to correct for the alignment of the detectors about the centre of the field of view. The raw data is then normalized with respect to the different detector efficiencies (see section on calibration). The raw data for opposing detectors is then merged to form 6 projections or merged arrays of size 128×22: i.e. since one line overlaps we have 22 not 24. An attenuation matrix is applied to each projection. A 17.5 cm diameter object is assumed and a constant attenuation co-efficient of 0.07 cm^{-1} used. Two smoothing filters are subsequently applied to each projection so that two images are eventually produced. The 'high resolution' image is smoothed in the horizontal direction only whereas the 'lower resolution' image is smoothed in the horizontal and vertical directions. Each of these corrected merged arrays is then convolved with a filter function derived from that given by Bracewell & Riddle (1967). This is applied to each of the 22 lines of each projection, the filter was initially applied in frequency space and is essentially a ramp, the amplification of frequencies being directly proportional to the frequency itself. However, rectilinear scan data consists of discrete elements rather than a continuous distribution. It is therefore convenient to apply the filter as a convolution of the data with the equivalent distribution in real space (Keyes 1976). Ideally an infinite number of terms is required in the convolution and modification to the filter function is necessary to allow for the finite number of terms available in the raw data. This modified convolution function was derived by iterative techniques using simulated data. The result of such a modification is to reduce the level of noise due to 'ringing' within the reconstructed image. Each filtered projection is rotated to its correct orientation and interpolated to give six 128 × 128 matrices. These six matrices, containing the filtered projections are then added together to form the final image. Subsequently the image is normalized to the total raw counts collected during the study and the data displayed as an image.

This filtering process is applied serially to both sets of smoothed raw data to yield both the 'high' and 'low' resolution images. Reconstruction time for each image is currently 2 minutes, i.e. 4 minutes for each slice.

IMAGE MANIPULATION

After an initial start up procedure in which it is necessary to access the computer via its own terminal, the entire process of data collection, reconstruction and display is under computer control and is interfaced to the user via the operator console. The computer systematically interrogates the console where all display and scanning parameters are selected. Images are displayed in pairs, a 'high' resolution (left) and a 'smoothed' image (right) as shown in Figure 4.6. For presentation purposes all image identification has been removed from the clinical examples; however, comprehensive documentation of scanning conditions is available as shown in Figure 4.6. Numerical values for PATIENT,

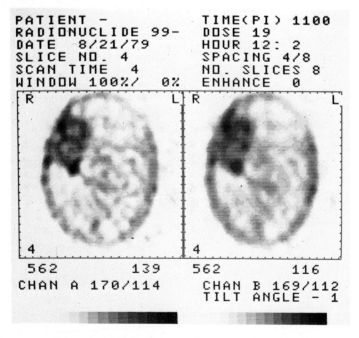

Fig. 4.6 Reconstructed image presentation complete with scanning parameters. High resolution reconstruction on the left, lower resolution reconstruction on the right.

TIME(PI)—post injection, RADIONUCLIDE and DOSE are obtained from the console via the numeric keypad. The DATE and TIME are taken directly from the computer real time clock. The SLICE NO., SPACING (inches), SCAN TIME (minutes), NO. SLICE (total number of slices requested in study) are read directly from the front panel switches. WINDOW refers to the upper and lower cut off values (as a percentage of the maximum count) used in the image display. The ENHANCE value indicates the modified grey scale assignment in the display and is shown as the grey scale at lower edge of image. An enhance value of zero (∅) gives a linear 16 level grey scale. Beneath each image the numerical value to the left indicates the total number of counts in the image ($\times 1000$). The right hand value gives the maximum pixel value. The TILT ANGLE (deg.) indicates the tilt applied to the gantry. CHAN A and CHAN B indicate the upper and lower energy window settings (keV). The two settings result from the fact that the machine is capable of allowing two distinct energy ranges. When the system is in this dual radionuclide mode the counts and positions for two distinct radionuclides located in the same region of the brain can be simultaneously recorded and reconstructed.

A facility has been provided which can be used to calibrate the response of the instrument to any pair of isotopes (Program DUIS). The procedure requires two scans of the ring phantom containing identical concentrations of each isotope, i.e. one scan for each of the isotopes to be imaged simultaneously. From these two images corrections are then determined for: (1) the scatter from each isotope into the energy window of the other, (2) the different sensitivities of the detector assemblies to each isotope, allowing equal concentrations of isotopes to be displayed at the same grey level. These corrections are automatically applied during image reconstruction.

After a set of slices has been collected and reconstructed various processing options are available using the computer terminal which has a conventional keyboard and printer. There are two basic programs; (a) OPTION which allows for the processing of the conventional transaxial slices and (b) LAT which allows reconstruction and processing of lateral view slices which are generated from the reconstructed transaxial slices.

The OPTION program allows the user to:

(1) Add or subtract reconstructed slices

Using this facility each transverse section image can be corrected for contributions derived from adjacent structures by subtracting appropriate proportions of adjacent slices.

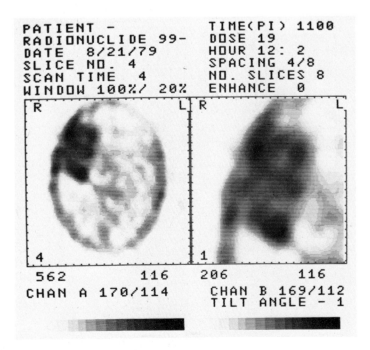

Fig. 4.7 Image manipulation—magnification.

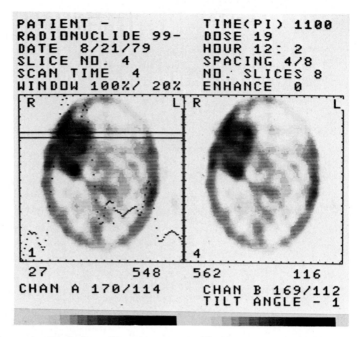

Fig. 4.8 Image manipulation—histogram output. Hardcopy output of the reconstructed count profile is also available.

(2) **Image magnification**

The facility of 'zooming a reconstructed slice' is also provided enabling any 64×64 area of the 128×128 image to be expanded to a full field display (Fig. 4.7).

(3) **Histogram plotting of the counts along any row or column of a reconstructed slice**

The user can select any vertical or horizontal line in a 128×128 image and determine the reconstructed value along that line. The slice is displayed on the console screen and a bright line is superimposed over the selected line for identification. A histogram is then superimposed over the slice (Fig. 4.8). The entire histogram is scaled to the maximum pixel value in the selected line. At the base of the display the maximum pixel value and the total number of counts in the selected line are displayed on the screen. The above procedure may be performed on a sum of lines in which case two bright lines are displayed identifying the first and last lines of the sum.

(4) **Selection of a variable shape region of interest (ROI) in a reconstructed slice**

Using this facility any region of the image can be outlined for digital and quantitative analysis (Fig. 4.9). This feature is implemented by displaying the slice on the screen, selecting the starting point and then moving a bug (bright spot on the screen) using the numeric keypad on the console to outline the region appropriately. When the region is closed, the following information is output on the console:

(a) Maximum pixel value in ROI.
(b) Maximum pixel value in slice.
(c) Total counts in ROI.
(d) Total counts in slice.

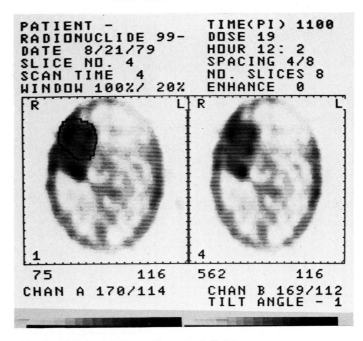

Fig. 4.9 Image manipulation—region of interest definition.

(e) Percentage of total slice counts in ROI.
(f) Number of pixels in ROI.
(g) Average ROI pixel count.

Further display facilities are provided allowing the manual display of slices with any desired parameter and also the ability to add comments to a displayed slice for photographic records.

Any display appearing on the television monitor can be recorded on X-ray or polaroid film using the photographic facilities provided from a high resolution slave monitor.

PERFORMANCE CHARACTERISTICS

The introduction of emission reconstruction tomography by Kuhl & Edwards (1963) also saw the advent of techniques to assess and measure parameters which will characterize the imaging capabilities of such instruments. It is necessary to consider the following physical parameters:

(a) Resolution within the plane of the slice.
(b) Slice width.
(c) Sensitivity of the detector assembly.
(d) The ability to quantify activity distributions.

(A) The measurement of the line spread function (LSF) within a slice

The LSF for ^{99m}Tc was measured using a phantom consisting of a circular perspex block, 20 cm in diameter and 5 cm thick, in which a series of 2.5 mm holes had been drilled in a spiral pattern. A short length of polyethylene tubing containing a solution of ^{99m}Tc (10 mCi/ml) was inserted into each hole in turn and 2 minute scans performed. This enabled the measurement of the LSF at known depths of scattering medium. An estimate of the full width at half

Table 4.1 FWHM and FWTM values for 'high' and 'low' resolution reconstructions on Cleon-710 imager

Reconstruction resolution	FWHM (mm)	FWTM (mm)
High	9.6 ± 0.2	15.4 ± 1.3
Low	11.5 ± 0.2	18.4 ± 1.2

maximum (FWHM) of the line spread function as a function of resolution elements was made using profiles through the reconstructed point source. The results are given in Table 4.1 and show the FWHM and FWTM (full width tenth maximum) for both the 'high' and 'low' resolution reconstructions. It should be noted that these values do not vary significantly across the field of view and that all points reconstruct as circles irrespective of their position within the field of view.

The use of a single FWHM value assumes that the system is linear and stationary and since the line spread function is not Gaussian it is not adequately defined by a single value.

(B) Measurement of slice thickness (FWHMs1)

The slice thickness is defined as the FWHM of the point spread function normal to the tomographic plane. Since the response is summed over a number of distances along the collimator axis a value for the thickness can only be derived from the reconstructed images. It is not simply a function of collimator response. It was measured by serially imaging a point source as it was moved along the axis perpendicular to the detection plane. A longitudinal profile was then obtained by plotting the counts within the region of the point source against distance.

A uniform slice thickness of 15 mm (FWHMs1) was found although it should be stressed that the response function is not rectangular in shape (Fig. 4.10). The tails do fall to zero but it is clear that data collection at 15 mm spacing of slices will result in considerable 'cross talk'.

It should be noted that the slice thickness is not simply a function of collimator response. In devices which rely on rotation or rotation and translation of a detector assembly at a fixed radius, the collimator characteristic alone will determine the slice thickness. (It is assumed that this is not affected by the

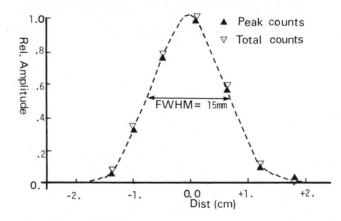

Fig. 4.10 Sensitivity distribution perpendicular to the plane of the slice—slice thickness (FWHMs1).

reconstruction process.) The result for these alternative single photon devices is to produce slices which have a concave (long focus detectors) or a convex (gamma cameras) cross section. The effect of a variable slice thickness is discussed in a later section.

(C) Measurement of sensitivity

Sensitivity is usually understood as that count rate obtained for a given activity concentration in a certain specified phantom. The phantom used was that defined by Kuhl et al (1976) i.e. a cylinder of 19 cm internal diameter and of 20 cm length. The walls were made of 0.5 cm thick perspex. Known amounts of activity were uniformly distributed within the cylinder and scanned using the recommended energy window for technetium of 130–170 keV. A value for the sensitivity of 15 600 counts μCi^{-1} ml^{-1} sec^{-1} was obtained. The value given was verified by reference to the raw counts thus removing any multiplicative factors occurring in the reconstruction. This cannot be stressed too highly since it has been found that manufacturers do not always normalize the reconstructed image values to the raw counts. The result may be a vastly increased value for the sensitivity of the instrument. This phenomenon existed on early software revisions of the Cleon-710 resulting in a value of 36 k counts μCi^{-1} ml^{-1} sec^{-1} using reconstructed counts. The definition used is not independent of the phantom, as self absorption within the phantom occurs. However, the cylindrical phantom would seem to give a value for the sensitivity which resembles that encountered in organ scanning; an advantage over more discrete source distributions.

A word of caution is in order as to the universal application of this parameter. The many different detector geometries now available make it difficult to estimate its role as a performance characteristic to measure detector efficiencies.

(D) Quantification

A major motivating force behind the introduction of emission computed tomography is its potential for quantifying radioisotope concentrations throughout a cross section. In an ideal environment the individual pixel values in an image should be directly proportional to radioisotope concentration in the corresponding element of the object (eqn. 1). Since the image pixels represent a volume in the object, expressions for activity per unit volume must be obtained.

$$[\mu Ci/cc]_{organ} = F[cts/pixel]_{image} \tag{1}$$

If F, the constant of proportionality can be obtained, then a solution exists. However, its derivation does not necessarily mean that it may be readily applied to clinical problems.

There are several sources of error inherent in emission tomographic imaging. Firstly gamma-ray detection equipment has a 'finite field of view', thus true line integrals are not recorded. This will have an effect, both in the plane of the section and in the plane perpendicular to it, i.e. the response must be independent of the source position within the field. Secondly, there is absorption within the medium containing the activity. Thirdly, there will be contributions from activity outside the field of view.

Within the plane of the slice, the error distribution seen in the reconstruction of a point source (Fig. 4.11) will exist at all points within an image. For large distributed sources this can be treated by subtraction of a constant background

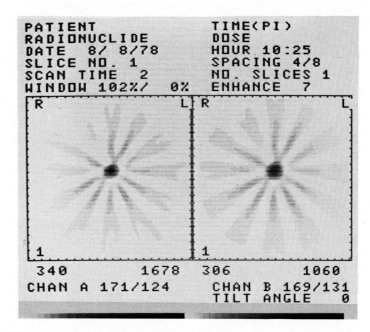

Fig. 4.11 Point source reconstruction with enhanced reconstruction artifacts.

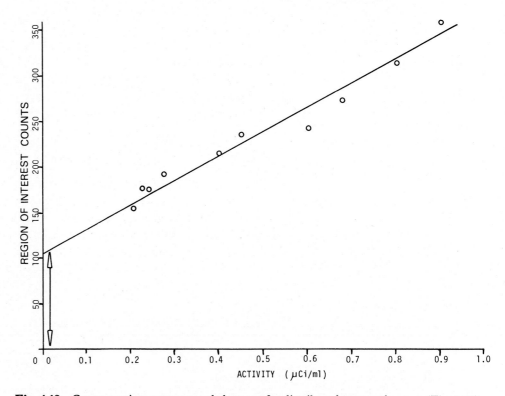

Fig. 4.12 Concentration versus recorded counts for distributed source phantom (Fig. 4.13).

component. However the structure of this noise component cannot be determined for more discrete source distributions since it is non-stationary and non-linear. This effect is demonstrated in Fig. 4.12. Each compartment within the phantom illustrated in Figure 4.13 was filled with known amounts of activity distributed at random. This was subsequently imaged, regions of interest drawn around each compartment (their size being equal to the compartment size) and

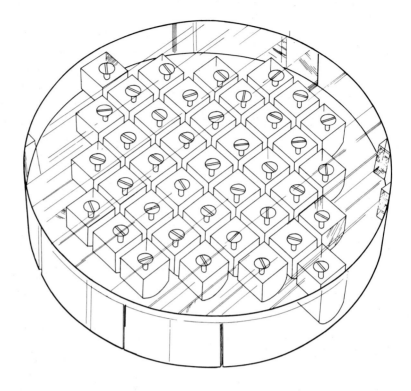

Fig. 4.13 Multihole phantom used to investigate quantitative aspects of Cleon-710.

the results plotted. A good correlation is obtained between counts and activity; however there is apparent activity (y intercept) at zero concentration, reflecting the large background contribution. This would not be observed if a single point source were imaged and consequently a different calibration factor would be obtained.

In order to achieve a high sensitivity detection device the Cleon-710 utilizes highly focussed detectors which necessarily have a wide angle of acceptance for emitted gamma-rays. As has been shown in a preceding section even with such detector geometry the reconstructed slices have a uniform slice thickness. This is important, since it allows extrapolation from areas in the reconstructed image to volume in the object to be done without a position dependent correction. This is not so with variable slice thickness detection systems (e.g. gamma cameras).

Correction for absorption of gamma-rays within the object is theoretically possible and using transmission scans of either X-ray or gamma-ray sources attenuation maps can be derived. Their application, however, is only possible where true line integrals are considered. The 'finite field of view' of the detectors has already been mentioned and the increased sensitivity so obtained is of obvious benefit. However if we consider a point in the plane of the slice, each of the detector pairs will observe that point at a different depth with consequently differing contributions from intervening activity, themselves subject to an unknown attenuation. The assumption is made that all detected activity results from emissions at the focus of the detector and that a single valued attenuation correction can be applied in each projection. This is clearly incorrect.

The current reconstruction nevertheless applies a constant attenuation correction to the raw data, assuming the brain to be an homogeneous absorbing medium. No account is taken of the source distribution, which, as has been shown, cannot be ignored. The problem has been recognized and iterative reconstruction techniques are being applied which allow the source distribution to be considered in the process of attenuation correction. This modification should lead to a significant improvement in image quantification than that currently available. This technique has been successfully applied by Budinger and Gullberg (1974) using a refinement of the technique to derive the actual shape of the attenuating volume prior to the final attenuation correction.

Provided that sufficient data is collected, contributions from activity outside the field of view can be eliminated. Since the sensitivity distribution perpendicular to the plane of the slice is known and constant it is possible to subtract the appropriate proportions of adjacent slices to correct for these contributions. This does imply that data collection protocols must allow for collection of data from at least three planes for a first order correction of a single plane.

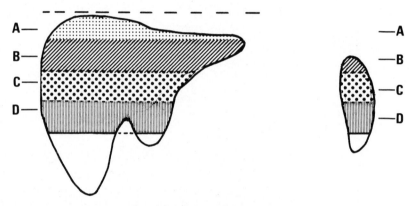

Fig. 4.14 Demonstration of 'partial volume effect' (see text).

When all these factors have been included it is still necessary to remember that patients are not phantoms. Distributions of activity within organs do not remain constant over large distances. Phantoms are usually designed so that their thickness is at least three times that of the slice FWHM. Where these extended distributions are not present 'partial volume effects' can be demonstrated. The result of the 'partial volume effect' is that fluctuations of activity which occur within dimensions less than approximately 2 × the FWHM of the resolution in the plane of, and perpendicular to, the slice are not accurately discernable. This effect is illustrated in Figure 4.14. If a uniform concentration of x μCi/ml is assumed for liver tissue and a concentration y μCi/ml for spleen then the values measured in slices A and D for liver would be less than x as would the concentration for spleen activity in slice B be less than y. Thus it is clear that without further information a single slice at A, B or D would result in an incorrect calculation or even diagnosis.

Although this illustrates the principle by reference to an entire organ, its implications for small 'cold' lesion detection is readily apparent. In the plane of the slice the point spread function acting around the circumference of a 'cold'

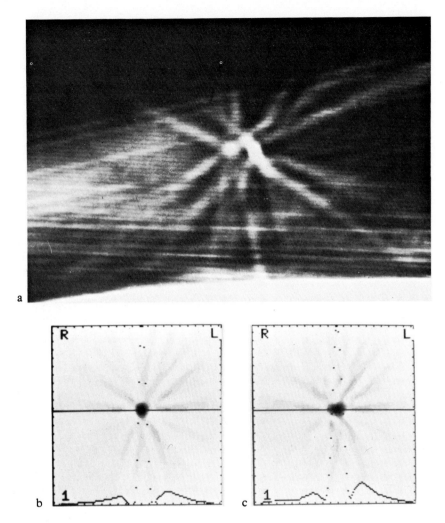

Fig. 4.15 (a) Reconstruction of a vibrating phantom using an X-ray transmission scanner.
(b) Reconstruction of stationary phantom using Cleon-710.
(c) Reconstruction of vibrating phantom using Cleon-710.
By courtesy of M. Flower, Royal Marsden Hospital, Sutton, England.

lesion will tend to 'fill in' the defect giving lower contrast (reduced lesion to organ ratio) and diminishing its size. Perpendicular to the slice the same phenomenon will occur since a large 'thin' lesion will be masked by activity from adjacent structures in the plane.

The implication for cold spot detection is that the slice thickness and reconstructed image resolution must be minimized within the limits of statistical fluctuations. This does not apply to hot spot detection. Provided the concentration of activity is sufficient to give a high target to background ratio, a 2 mm lesion can be seen by an instrument with 2 cm resolution. Again an accurate assessment of its size and of its true activity concentration is difficult.

PATIENT MOVEMENT

The unique data collection system of the Cleon-710 does significantly reduce the errors incurred by patient movement. Figure 4.15 (a) demonstrates the effect which is observed when an attenuating object is moved cyclically between two points 25 times per minute in a transmission tomographic system. Star pattern artifacts are observed and the object tends to be reconstructed as two distinct objects. In comparison Figure 4.15 (b & c) shows the result when the attenuating medium is replaced by a radioactive source. Figure 4.15 (b) shows the source without motion, Figure 4.15 (c) with motion. A profile through the source has been superimposed on each image. The counts displayed below the image refer to the profiles. The left hand number is the total count under the profile ($\times 1000$), the right hand number is the peak value. The reconstruction shows no artifacts due to motion. The profiles indicate that although the resolution has decreased there has been no significant change in sensitivity with values of 103 000 and 102 000 for the total profile count.

CONCLUSION

The Cleon-710 tomographic brain scanner has proven its clinical value. It has good performance characteristics in terms of spatial resolution and sensitivity. It is feasible to improve the collimator detector response (without significant loss of spatial resolution) in order to gain at least a 2 fold increase in sensitivity. This could lead to scanning times of 60 seconds/slice. In our experience of 2 years with this device, it has proven itself as a very reliable instrument, with good mechanical and electrical stability (down time of less than 5 per cent). It has been operated (within the clinical environment) by radiographers and technicians.

REFERENCES

Bracewell R N, Riddle A C 1967 Inversion of fan beam scans in radio-astronomy. Astrophysical Journal 150: 427–434
Budinger T F, Gullberg G T 1974 Three-dimensional reconstruction of isotope distributions. Physics in Medicine and Biology 10: 387–380
Keyes W I 1976 A practical approach to transverse-section gamma-ray imaging. British Journal of Radiology 49: 62–70
Kuhl D E, Edwards R Q 1974 Image separation radioisotope scanning. Radiology 80: 653–661
Kuhl D E et al 1976 The Mark IV System for radionuclide computed tomography of the brain. Radiology 121: 405–413

5. THE CLEON-711 TOMOGRAPHIC BODY IMAGER

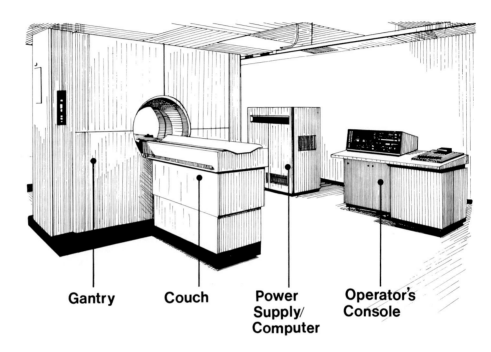

Gantry   Couch   Power Supply/ Computer   Operator's Console

Fig. 5.1 The Cleon-711 Tomographic Body Imager.

This device is currently under evaluation at two centres, one in Europe (at the Middlesex Hospital Medical School) and the other in the United States of America. Its appearance (see Fig. 5.1) and mode of operation resembles that of the Cleon-710 brain imager discussed in the previous chapter. Only those aspects which differ significantly from the Cleon-710 imager will be presented in this chapter. The Cleon-711 imager is currently in development and the reader is advised that the information and results given are those available at the time of writing (September, 1979) with the machine at the prototype stage.

PRINCIPLES OF OPERATION

The gantry assembly contains ten detector assemblies which scan an aperture of 60 cm diameter. The detector assemblies are essentially identical to those described for the Cleon-710, except that improved shielding has increased the upper energy limit to approximately 370 keV. The focussing collimators have a focal length of approximately 42.5 cm, with a FWHM (full width at half maximum) of 1.7 cm in the plane of the slice and 2.0 cm perpendicular to the slice. The detectors are mounted in a clockwise fashion around the opening at 36° separation. Figure 5.2 illustrates the pairwise motion of the detectors. When

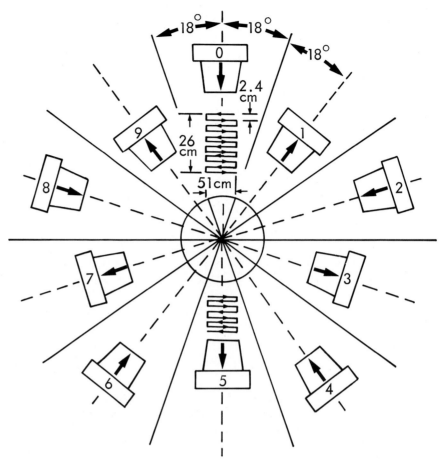

Fig. 5.2 Diagrammatic representation of the paired motion of the detectors of the Cleon-711.

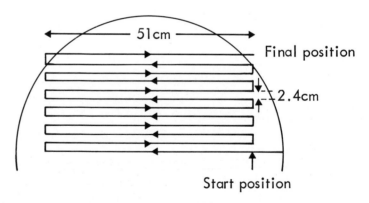

Fig. 5.3 Scan pattern of the focal point of a single detector assembly.

one detector is scanning across and moving toward the opening, the opposite detector is traversing in the opposite direction and moving away from the opening. Whilst acquiring data for a slice, each detector scans 12 lines with a spacing of 2.4 cm, the focal point of the detector scans through half of the field of view (Fig. 5.3). The data from opposing pairs of detectors is combined to form a raster scan over the entire field of view. When each detector has scanned 12 lines, it will have sampled an angle of 18°, this gives a total of 180° for the ten detectors. To complete the full angular sampling, the entire detector assembly is rotated 18° counter-clockwise and the scanning operation repeated with the detectors returning to the start positions. The gantry is finally rotated 18° clockwise to complete the cycle. This sequence is illustrated in Figure 5.4. Once such a scanning sequence has been initiated from the operator console, the motion of the detectors and patient couch are under computer control with up to 8 slices being scanned automatically. Increments up to 4.5 cm, in multiples of 3 mm, can be selected for the slice spacing, with a fixed scanning time of 5 minutes. The gantry can be tilted up to ±15° from the vertical to facilitate viewing sections of the body at the appropriate angle.

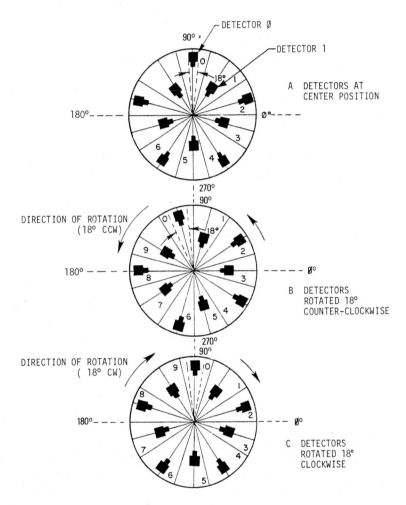

Fig. 5.4 The gantry rotation sequence of the Cleon-711 imager.

The collection and transmission of data to the computer is as described in the previous chapter. Each scan line, length 51 cm, is divided into 128 resolution elements, giving a pixel element length of 4 mm. In order to image better small organs, such as the brain, a half field mode has been provided in which the scanned field of view is reduced to 21.5 cm. Although the detectors scan as described, an initial offset is applied such that only the central 21.5 cm of the full field scan line is used. Twelve such scan lines are performed, each with 128 resolution elements, which scan the full radius of the field of view. A raster element length of 1.68 mm is thus obtained. A 128 × 128 image is reconstructed in each case.

GANTRY CALIBRATION

As previously described, careful quality control of the centre of rotation is essential for artifact free reconstructions. Unlike the Cleon-710 the offsets, which correct for focal length variations in the detector assemblies, have been incorporated in the mechanical alignment of the gantry. The calculation of the offset values which correct for the lateral displacement of the focal point relative to the mechanical centre of the innermost line has been automated. Four scans of a manufacturer supplied line source calibration phantom are recorded. A computer program then minimizes the displacement between the images in the central line scans from opposing pairs of detectors, using an average of the four scans. These twenty correction values, one for each detector at each gantry position, are subsequently applied to the raw data during image reconstruction.

Routine peaking of the individual detectors is accomplished using a ring source centred in the gantry. The detectors are positioned equidistant from the centre (the CAL position) and small adjustments to the individual high voltage supplies made via a calibration box in the gantry. For ^{99m}Tc and ^{57}Co, a comparison is made between the counts recorded in two narrow (5 keV) windows, which incorporate the rising and falling edges of the photopeak. High voltage adjustments are made to give a zero difference between the counts recorded in the two windows. For other isotopes, spectra have to be plotted manually to ascertain the correct window settings and it is assumed that the relative positions of the photopeaks from each detector is maintained at these energies.

IMAGE RECONSTRUCTION AND DISPLAY

The steps involved in image reconstruction are identical to those described for the Cleon-710 brain imager. However, the input data consists of 10 merged arrays (5 arrays at each gantry position) each of 128×22 elements. In the current version of the software the user is able to vary the diameter over which a constant absorption correction is applied. The instrument assumes that the object is circularly symmetric and centred in the gantry opening. It is possible by selecting an appropriate value for the diameter to remove the attentuation correction. As previously discussed it is not possible to apply an attentuation correction without reference to the source distribution. The assumption about object shape and attenuation characteristic cannot be considered as valid especially for body imaging. Reconstructed images are presented in pairs and can be manipulated from the operator console to obtain the desired display. The user can modify the background cut-off, and saturation level assignment (all values above a selected percentage of the maximum image pixel are displayed at maximum intensity) and the grey scale assignment for the display. Hardcopy output is provided on 10×8 in X-ray film, polaroid, or print output using a Vidicam copier. Storage of raw or reconstructed image data is available on floppy disc. This data can be interrogated further using the computer terminal. The programs OPTION, LAT and DUIS allow the user to perform those functions previously described for the Cleon-710 imager.

PERFORMANCE CHARACTERISTICS

(a) Line spread response function in the plane of the slice

Measurements were made in both the full and half field modes using the

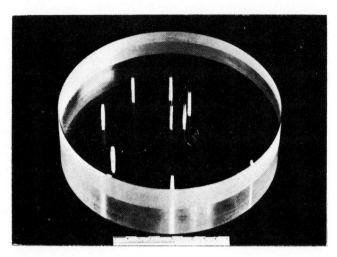

Fig. 5.5 Phantom used to determine the line spread response function in half field mode.

phantom described in the preceding chapter (see Fig. 5.5). For the full field analysis, a perspex phantom 45 cm in diameter was used whilst a standard 20 cm diameter phantom was used for the half field mode. The results are given in Table 5.1. The values for FWHM and FWTM are 23.6 mm and 41.2 mm for the full field mode and 14.3 mm and 27.3 mm for the half field mode.

Table 5.1 Line spread response characteristics in the plane of the slice for the Cleon-711 imager

| Mode | Resolution | |
	FWHM (mm) (Full width at half maximum)	FWTM (mm) (Full width at tenth maximum)
Full field	23.6 ± 1.7	41.2 ± 2.2
Half field	14.3 ± 1.2	27.3 ± 1.6

(b) Measurement of slice thickness

An estimate of the FWHM and FWTM of the slice width was made using a point source placed at various depths within a 45 cm diameter perspex block for the full field mode and a 20 cm diameter absorber for the half field mode. A series of images was obtained for both modes by moving a point source along the axis perpendicular to the detection plane. A fixed region of interest surrounding the reconstructed point source was used to obtain the counts in each image. These were then plotted to give a profile of activity against distance, from which the parameters were calculated. The values obtained are given in Table 5.2.

Table 5.2 Slice thickness values for the Cleon-711 imager

| Mode | Slice thickness | |
	FWHM (mm) (Full width at half maximum)	FWTM (mm) (Full width at tenth maximum)
Full field	20.6 ± 0.7	46.8 ± 1.0
Half field	21.7 ± 0.8	38.6 ± 2.3

(c) Detector sensitivity measurements

The standard phantom described, a cylinder of 19 cm internal diameter and of length 20 cm, was used to determine the sensitivity in both full and half field

Table 5.3 Sensitivity values for the Cleon-711 tomographic body imager

Energy range	Sensitivity counts μCi^{-1} ml^{-1} sec^{-1}	
	Full field	Half field
115–170 keV	5678.6	10 436.8
130–170 keV	3933.5	7253.3

modes. The values obtained are dependent on the energy window settings. The results presented in Table 5.3 give values for two energy ranges:

(i) At the manufacturer's recommended settings of 130–170 keV, which is an asymmetric window. Such a window is usually chosen to exclude scattered radiation, which if included will tend to degrade the image.

(ii) With the energy window at 115–170 keV. This is a less asymmetric window including more scattered radiation but which does not seem to degrade the image. There is no loss of spatial resolution, but there is a significant increase in sensitivity with a concommitant decrease in statistical noise in the reconstructed image.

In such a data collection system, the sensitivity measured is not equivalent to a static measurement of detector sensitivity. For a significant portion of the scanning time, the detectors are not collecting data, e.g., during detector motion between scan lines. Also, the focal point of a particular detector only traverses the region of the source for between 25 per cent and 50 per cent of the scanning time, depending on the mode of operation. The amount of time actually spent collecting data will depend on the size of object being scanned, reflecting the fact that any sensitivity measurement will be phantom dependent.

CONCLUSION

The Cleon-711 tomographic imager offers one approach to the problem of transverse section imaging in the body. Like the Cleon-710 its detection geometry means that the reconstructed image is not susceptible to artifacts due to patient or organ movement. However the partial volume effect outlined previously will be of greater significance due to the increased slice width and image resolution by comparison with those characteristics of other techniques. Slice thickness can only be changed by new collimators. The current image resolution does not represent the full potential of the instrument since the limit of resolution is that of the collimators i.e. 18 mm c.f. a currently measured value of 24 mm. A fixed scanning time is an obvious limitation. Although it does not seem possible to decrease this time, longer scan times would be valuable in imaging organs with low radiotracer uptake.

The effect of decreased sensitivity and resolution of the Cleon-711 compared with the brain imager can only be made from its clinical efficacy. Such a judgement cannot be made from physical measurements alone.

Bibliography

Akcasu A Z et al 1974 Coded aperture gamma-ray imaging with stochastic apertures. Optical Engineering 13:117

Anger H O 1966 The scintillation camera for radioisotope localization. In: Hoffman G, Sheer K E (eds) Radioisotope in der Lokalisation–diagnostik. Schattauer, Stuttgart, pp 1–21

Anger H O 1968 Tomographic gamma-ray scanner with simultaneous readout of several planes. In: Gottschalk A, Beck R N (eds) Fundamental problems in scanning. Thomas, Springfield, Ill., pp 195–211

Anger H 1973 Multiple plane tomographic scanner. In: Freedman G S (ed) Tomographic imaging in nuclear medicine. Soc Nucl Med, New York, pp 2–15

Baron J C, Comar D, Bousser M G, Soussaline F, Crouzel C, Kellershohn C, Castaigne P 1978 Etude tomographique chez l'homme, du débit sanguin et de la consommation d'oxygène du cerveau par inhalation continue d'oxygène 15. Rev. Neurol. (Paris) 134: 545–556

Barrett H 1972 Fresnel zone plate imaging in nuclear medicine. J Nucl Med 13: 382–385

Barrett H H, Horrigan F A 1973 Fresnel zone plate imaging of gamma rays. Appl Optics: 2686–2701

Barrett H H, Bowen T, Herschel R S, Gordon S K, De Lise D A 1975 Noise and dose considerations in transaxial tomography with X-ray and particles. In: Imaging processing for 2D and 3D reconstruction from projections; Theory and practice in medicine and the physical sciences. Optical Soc of Am WB2–1, Stanford, Calif.

Bates R H T, Peters T M 1971 Towards improvements in tomography. New Zealand J Sci 14: 883–896

Beattie J W 1975 Tomographic reconstruction from fan beam geometry using Radon's integration method. IEEE Trans Nucl Sci NS-22(1): 359–363

Berger G, Mazière M, Marazano C, Comar D 1978 Carbon 11 labelling of the psychoactive drug O-methyl-bufornine and its distribution in the animal organism. Eur J Nucl Med 3: 101–104

Berry M V, Gibbs D F 1970 The interpretation of optical projections. Proc R Soc Lond 314: 143–152

Bocage E M 1974 Patent No. 536,464, Paris France. Quoted in Massiot J: History of tomography. Medica Mundi 19: 106–115

Bowley A R, Taylor C G, Causer D A, et al 1973 A radioisotope scanner for rectilinear, arc, transverse section and longitudinal section scannings: ASS-the Aberdeen Section Scanner. Br J Radiol 46: 262–271

Boyd D, Coonrod J, Dehnert J, et al 1974 High-pressure xenon proportional chamber for X-ray laminographic reconstruction using fan-beam geometry. IEEE Trans Nucl Sci NS-21(1): 184–187

Bracewell R N 1956 Strip integration in radioastronomy. Aust J Phys 9: 198–217

Bracewell R N 1958 Radio interferometry of discrete sources. Proceedings of the Institute of Radio Engineers 46: 97–105

Bracewell R N 1965 The Fourier transform and its applications. McGraw–Hill, New York

Bracewell R N, Riddle A C 1967 Inversion of fan-beam scans in radio astronomy. Astrophys J 150: 427–434

Brigham E O 1974 The fast fourier transform. Prentice-Hall, Englewood Cliffs, N.J, p 113

Brooks R A, Di Chiro G 1975 Theory of image reconstruction in computed tomography. Radiology 117: 561–572

Brooks R A, Di Chiro G 1976 Statistical limitations in x-ray reconstructive tomography. Med Phys 3: 237–240

Brooks R A, Di Chiro G 1976 Principles of computer assisted tomography (CAT) in radiographic and radioisotopic imaging. Phys Med Biol 21: 689–732

Brown C 1974 Multiplex imaging with multiple pinhole cameras. J Appl Phys: 1806–1811

Brownell G L, Burnham C A 1973 In: Freedman G S (ed) Tomographic imaging in nuclear medicine. Soc Nucl Med, New York, pp 154–164

Brownell G L, Burnham C A 1973 MGH positron camera. In: Tomographic imaging in nuclear medicine. Soc Nucl Med, New York, p 154

Brownell G L, Burnham C A, Chesler D A, et al 1977 Transverse section imaging of radionuclide distributions in heart, lung and brain. In: Ter Pogossian M M, Phelps M E, Brownell G L, et al (eds) Reconstruction tomography in diagnostic radiology and nuclear medicine. University Park Press, Baltimore, pp 293–307

Brownell G L, Burnham C A, Hoop B Jr 1973 Positron scintigraphy with short-lived cyclotron produced radiopharmaceuticals. In: Medical radioisotope scintigraphy. IAEA, Vienna, vol 1, pp 313–330

Brownell G L, Burnham C A, Wilensky S, Aronow S, Kazemi S, Strieder D 1968 New developments in positron scintigraphy and the application of cyclotron produced positron emitters. Medical radioisotope scintigraphy, Proc Symp. Salzburg (1968). IAEA, Vienna, vol 1, pp 163–176

Brownell G L, Correia J A, Zamenhof R G 1978 Positron instrumentation. In: Lawrence J H, Budinger T F (eds) Recent advances in nuclear medicine, vol 5, Grune & Stratton, New York, pp 1–49

Budinger T F, Gulberg G T 1974 Three-dimensional reconstruction in nuclear medicine by iterative least square and Fourier transform techniques. Lawrence Berkeley Laboratory LBL–2146

Budinger T F, Gullberg G T 1974 Three-dimensional reconstruction in nuclear medicine emission imaging. IEEE Trans Nucl Sci NS21(3): 2–20

Budinger T F, Gullberg G T 1974 Three-dimensional reconstruction of isotope distribution. Phys Med Biol 19: 387–389

Budinger T F, Gullberg G T 1977 Transverse section reconstruction of gamma ray emitting radionuclides in patients. In: Ter Pogossian M M (ed) Reconstruction tomography in diagnostic radiology and nuclear medicine. University Park Press, Baltimore, p 315

Budinger T F, Harpootlian J 1975 Transverse section reconstruction from multiple gamma-camera views using frequency filtering. Lawrence Berkeley Laboratory Report No LBL 2862

Budinger T F, MacDonald B 1975 Reconstruction of the Fresnel-coded gamma camera images by digital computer. J Nucl Med 16: 309–313

Budinger T F, Gullberg G T, Huesman R H 1979 Emission computed tomography in image reconstruction from projections: implementation and appreciation. Herman G (ed) Springer-Verlag, New York

Budinger T F, Cahoon J L, Derenzo S E, et al 1977 Three-dimensional imaging of the myocardium with radionuclides. Radiology 125: 433–439

Budinger T F, Derenzo S E, Gullberg G T, Greenberg W L, Huesman R H 1976 Emission computed axial tomography. LBL–4794 IAEA–SM–210/124

Budinger T F, Derenzo S E, Greenberg W, Gullberg G T, Huesman R H 1978 Quantitative potentials of dynamic emission computed tomography. J Nucl Med 19: 309–315

Budinger T F, Derenzo S E, Gullberg G T, et al 1977 Emission computer assisted tomography with single-photon and positron annihilation photon emitters. J Comput Assist Tomogr 1: 131–145

Budinger T F, Gullberg G T, Moyer B K, Cahoon J L, Huesman R H 1976 Transverse section imaging of the myocardium. J Nucl Med 17: 552

Burdine J A, Murphy P H, De Puey E G 1979 Radionuclide computed tomography of the body using routine radiopharmaceuticals in clinical applications. J Nucl Med 20: 108–114

Chang L T 1978 A method for attenuation correction in radionuclide computed tomography. IEEE Trans Nucl Sci No NS–25, p 638

Chang L T 1979 Attenuation correction and incomplete projection in single photon emission computed tomography. IEEE Trans Nucl Sci Ns–26, 2, 2780

Chang L T, MacDonald B, Perez-Mendez V, Shiraiski L 1975 Coded aperture imaging of gamma-rays using multiple pinhole arrays and multiwire proportional chamber detector. IEEE Trans Nucl Sci NS–22, No 1

Chesler D A 1972 Positron tomography and three-dimensional reconstruction techniques. Proc Symp Radionucl Tomog. New York

Chesler D A 1973 Positron tomography and three-dimensional reconstruction technique. In: Freedman G S (ed) Tomographic imaging in nuclear medicine. Soc Nucl Med, New York, pp 176–183

Chesler D A, Riederer S J 1975 Ripple suppression during reconstruction in transverse tomography. Phys Med Biol 20: 632–636

Chesler D A, Riederer S J, Pelc N J 1977 Noise due to photon counting statistics in computed x-ray tomography. J Comput Assist Tomogr 1: 64–74

Chesler D A, Aronow S, Correll J E, et al 1977 Statistical properties and simulation studies of transverse section algorithms. In: Ter Pogossian M M, Phelps M E, Brownell G L, et al (eds) Reconstruction tomography in diagnostic radiology and nuclear medicine. University Park Press, Baltimore, pp 49–58

Chesler D A, Hales C, Anatowitch O J, Hoop B 1975 Three-dimensional reconstruction of lung perfusion images with positron detectors. J Nucl Med 16: 80

Cho Z H, Ahn I S 1975 Computer algorithm for the tomographic image reconstruction with x-ray transmission scans. Comput Biomed Res 8: 8–25

Cho Z H, Furukhi M R 1977 Bismuth germanate as a potential scintillation detector in positron cameras. J Nucl Med 18: 840–844

Cho Z H, Chan J K, Eriksson L 1976 Circular ring transverse axial positron camera for three-dimensional reconstruction of radionuclide distribution. IEEE Trans Nucl Sci NS–23

Cho Z H, Cohen M B, Singh M 1977 Performance and evaluation of the circular ring transverse axial positron camera (CRTAPC). IEEE Nucl Sci NS 24: 530–543

Cho Z H, Nalciglu O, Faruki M R 1978 Analysis of a cylindrical hybrid positron camera with bismuth germanate (BGO) scintillation crystals. IEEE NS 25: 952–963

Cho Z H, Chan J K, Hall E L, et al 1975 A comparative study of 3-D image reconstruction algorithms with reference to number of projections and noise filtering. IEEE Trans Nucl Sci NS-22(1): 344–358

Cho Z H, Chan J K, Eriksson L, et al 1975 Positron ranges obtained from biomedically important positron emitting radionuclides. J Nucl Med 16: 1174

Chong L T 1978 A method for attenuation correction in radionuclide computed tomography. IEEE Trans Nucl Sci 638–643

Clocker E F, Zimmerman R A, Phelps M E, et al 1976 The effect of steroids on the extravascular distribution of radiographic contrast material and Technetium-pertechnetate in brain tumours as determined by computed tomography. Radiology 119: 471–474

Comar D, Mazièrè M, Berger G, Mestelan G 1976 Quelques exemples de l'intérêt des molécules marquées au ^{11}C en recherche médicale. BIST 220, 19–26

Cormack A M 1963 Representation of a function by its line integrals, with some radiological applications. J Appl Phys 34: 2722–2727

Cormack A M 1964 Representation of a function by its line integrals with some radiological applications. II J Appl Phys 35: 2908–2913

Cormack A M 1973 Reconstruction of densities from their projections, with applications in radiological physics. Phys Med Biol 18: 195–207

Crouzel C, Comer D, Berger G, Mazière M, Soussaline F, Todd-Pokropek A E, Baron J C, Guenard H, Verhas M 1978 First clinical results using short lived radioisotopes produced by a medical cyclotron. In: VIIIth Int. Conf on Cyclotrons and their medical applications. Bloomington

Crowther R A, Klug A 1974 Three-dimensional image reconstruction on an extended field—a fast stable algorithm. Nature (Lond) 252: 490–492

Crowther R A, DeRosier D J, Klug A 1970 The reconstruction of a three-dimensional structure from projections and its application to electron microscopy. Prod R Soc Lond 317: 319–340

Dehnert J, Boyd D 1973 A comparison study of some computer reconstruction techniques. High Energy Physics Lab Rep 276, Stanford Univ, Stanford

Dendy P P, McNais J W, MacDonald A F, et al 1977 An evaluation of transverse axial emission tomography of the brain in the clinical situation. Br J Radiol 50: 555–561

Derenzo S E 1977 Positron ring cameras for emission computed tomography. IEEE NS 24: 811–885

Derenzo S E, Budinger T F, Cahoon J L, et al 1977 High resolution computed tomography of positron emitters, IEEE NS 24: 544–558

Derenzo S E, Zaklad H, Budinger T F, et al 1975 Analytical study of a high-resolution positron ring detector system for transaxial reconstruction tomography. J Nucl Med 16: 1166–1173

DeRosier D J, Klug A 1968 Reconstruction of three-dimensional structures from electron micrographs. Nature (Lond) 217: 130–134

Eichling J O, Higgins C S, Ter Pogossian M M 1977 Determination of radionuclide concentrations with positron CT scanning (PETT): Concise communication. J Nucl Med 18: 845–847

Ein-gal M 1974 The shadow transform: An approach to cross-sectional imaging. Tech Rep 6581-1, Information Systems Lab, Stanford Univ, Stanford

Ell P J, Jarritt P H, Deacon J, Brown N J G, Williams E S 1978 Emission computerized tomography. A new diagnostic imaging technique. The Lancet 2: 608–610

Ell P J, Jarritt P H, Langford R, Pearce P 1979 Is there a future for single photon emission tomography? RÖFO, 130, 4, 499–507

Eriksson L, Cho Z H 1976 Absorption correction in positron (annihilation gamma coincidence detection) transverse axial tomography. Phy Med Biol 21: 429–433

Eriksson L, Widen L, Bergstrom M, et al 1978 Evaluation of a high resolution ring detector positron camera system. J Comput Assist Tomogr 2: 649–650

Flower M A, Parker R P, Coles I P, Fox R A, Trott N G 1978 Feasibility of absolute activity measurements using the Cleon emission tomography system. Presented at the Annual

Meeting of the Radiological Society of North America, as a work-in-progress report

Freedman G S 1973 Tomographic imaging in nuclear medicine. Soc Nucl Med, New York

Friedman M I, Beattie J W, Laughlin J S 1974 Cross-sectional absorption density reconstruction for treatment planning. Phys Med Biol 19: 819–830

Gaarder N T, Herman GT 1972 Algorithms for reproducing objects from their x-rays. Comput Graph Image Process 1: 97–106

Genna S, Pang S C, Burrows B A 1976 Analysis of an accurate gamma camera for transaxial reconstruction. In: Medical radionuclide imaging. Proc Symp IAEA, Los Angeles

Gilbert P F C 1972 The reconstruction of a three-dimensional structure from projections and its application to electron microscopy. II Direct methods. Proc R Soc Lond [Biol] 182: 89–102

Gilbert P F C 1972 Iterative methods for the reconstruction of three-dimensional objects from projections. J Theor Biol 36: 105–117

Goitein M 1972 Three-dimensional density reconstructions from a series of two-dimensional projections. Nucl Instr Meth 101: 509–513

Gold B, Rader C M 1969 In digital processing of signals. McGraw-Hill, New York, pp 226–232

Gordon R, Herman G T 1974 Three-dimensional reconstruction from projections: A review of algorithms. International Review of Cytology 38: 111–151

Gordon R, Bender R, Herman G T 1970 Algebraic reconstruction techniques (ART) for three-dimensional electron microscopy and x-ray photography. J Theor Biol 29: 471

Gough P T, Bates R H T 1972 Computer generated holograms for processing radiographic data. Comput Biomed Res 5: 700–708

Grant D 1972 Tomosynthesis: A three-dimensional radiographic imaging technique. IEEE Trans Biomed Eng BME–19 No 1

Hanson K M, Boyd D P 1978 The characteristics of computed tomographic reconstruction noise and their effect on detectability. IEEE Trans Nucl Sci 25: 160–163

Harper P V 1968 The three-dimensional reconstruction of isotope distributions. Fundamental problems in scanning. C C Thomas, Springfield, Ill

Herman G T et al 1975 Bayesian and convolution type algorithms for divergent and parallel x-ray beams. In: Workshop on reconstruction tomography in diagnostic radiology and nuclear medicine, San Juan, Apr 17–19

Herman G T, Lakshminarayanan A V, Naparstek A 1976 Convolution reconstruction techniques for divergent beams. Comp Biol Med 6: 259–271

Herman G T, Rowland S 1973 Three methods for reconstructing objects from x-rays: a comparative study. Comp Graph Image Process 2: 151–178

Hill T C, Còstello P, Gramm H F, McNeil B J 1978 Preliminary observation of the clinical value of emission computed tomography. J Nucl Med 19: 684

Hoffman E J, Phelps M E 1976 An analysis of some of the physical aspects of positron transaxial tomography. Compu Bio Med 6: 345–360

Hoffman E J, Huang S C, Phelps M E 1979 Quantitation in positron emission computed tomography: 1 Effect of object size. J Comput Assist Tomogr 3(3): 299–308

Hoffman E J, Phelps M E, Mullani N et al 1976 Design and performance characteristics of a whole body positron transaxial tomograph. J Nucl Med 17: 493–502

Hoffman E J, Weiss E S, Phelps M E et al Transaxial tomographic imaging of canine myocardium with ^{11}C-palmitic acid. J Nucl Med (in press)

Hounsfield G N 1968 A method of and apparatus for examination of a body by radiation such as x- or gamma-radiation. British Patent No 12839 15, London, 1972. Issued to EMI Ltd. Application filed Aug

Hounsfield G N 1973 Computerized transverse axial scanning (tomography): Part 1 Description of system. Br J Radiol 46: 1016–1022

Hsieh R C, Wee W G 1976 On methods of three-dimensional reconstruction from a set of radioisotope scintigrams. IEEE Trans on systems. Man and Cybernetics SNC-6, 12: 854

Huesman R H 1966 The effects of a finite number of projection angles and finite lateral sampling of projections on the propagation of statistical errors in transverse section reconstruction. Lawrence Berkeley Laboratory Report LBL-4773

Huesman R H 1975 Analysis of statistical errors for transverse section reconstruction. Lawrence Berkeley Laboratory Report LBL–4278, Univ Calif

Huesman R H 1977 Medical radionuclide imaging. IAEA, Vienna

Huesman R H 1977 The effects of a finite number of projection angles and finite lateral sampling of projections on the propagation of statistical errors in transverse section reconstruction. Phys Med Biol 22: 511–521

Jacobi C G J 1846 Über ein leichtes Verfahren die in der Theorie der Säculärstörungen vorkommenden Gleichungen numerisch aufzulösen. Crelle J 30: 51–94

Jarritt P H, Ell P J, Myers M, Brown N J G, Deacon J M 1979 A new transverse section brain imager for single-gamma emitters. J Nucl Med 20: 319–327

Jaszczak R J, Chang L T, Murphy P H 1979 Single photon emission computed tomography using multi-slice fan beam collimators. IEEE Trans Nucl Sci NS–26

Jaszczak R J, Murphy P H, Huard D 1977 Radionuclide emission computed tomography of the head with ^{99m}Technetium and a scintillation camera. J Nucl Med 18: 373

John F 1955 Plane waves and spherical means applied to partial differential equations. Wiley Interscience, New York

Johnson S A 1975 Reconstruction of acoustic velocity cross sections from multiangular ultrasonic scans. Bull Am Phys Soc 20: 542

Jones T, Chesler D A, Ter Pogossian M M 1976 The continuous inhalation of oxygen 15 for assessing regional oxygen extraction in the brain of man. Br J Radiol 49: 339–343

Jordan K, Friel H-J, Gettner U, Kaempf E, Geisler S, Harsdorf J v, Nentwig C 1974 A new concept of an experimental tomographic scanner. 1st World Congress of Nucl Med. Tokyo, Proceedings, p 1274

Junginger H G, van Haeringen W 1972 Calculation of three-dimensional reflective-index field using phase integrals. Optics commun 5: 1–4

Kay D B, Keyes J W, Simon W 1974 Radionuclide tomographic image reconstruction using Fourier transform techniques. J Nucl Med 15: 981–986

Kay D B, Keys J W 1975 First order corrections for absorption and resolution compensation in radionuclide Fourier tomography. J Nucl Med 16: 540

Keyes W I 1976 Current status of single photon emission computerized tomography IEEE Trans Nucl Sci No 26, 2 April, p 2752

Keyes W I 1976 A practical approach to transverse section gamma ray imaging. Br J Radiol 49: 62–70

Keyes W I, Barber D C, Mallard J R 1973 Quantitative multi-level display of scan data via a small digital computer. Phys Med Biol 18: 133–137

Keyes J W, Leonard P F, Svetkoff D J et al 1978 Myocardial imaging using emission computed tomography. Radiology 127: 809–812

Keyes J W, Kay D B, Simon W 1973 Radionuclide three dimensional spatial imaging. Invest Radiol 8: 277–178

Keyes J W, Chesser R, Undrill P E 1976 Transverse-section emission tomography. 7th L H Gray Conference: Medical images: Formation, perception and measurements. Wiley, New York pp 51–67

Keyes J W, Kay D B, Lees D E B et al 1977 Applied comparisons of methods for radionuclide transverse section tomography. In: Proc 1st World Congress in Nucl Med, p 1281–1283

Keyes et al 1977 The humongotron—a scintillation camera transaxial tomograph. J Nucl Med 18: 381–387

Kircos L T, Leonard P F, Keyes J W 1978 An optimized collimator for single photon computed tomography with a scintillation camera. J Nucl Med 19: 322–323

Klug A, Crowther R A 1972 Three-dimensional image reconstruction from the viewpoint of information theory. Nature (Lond) 238: 435

Knoll G F, Williams J J 1977 Application of a ring pseudorandom aperture for transverse section tomography. IEEE Trans Nucl Sci NS–24. No 1

Koehler A M, Dickinson J G, Preston W M 1965 Radiat Res 26: 335

Koral K F, Rogers W L, Knoll G F 1975 Digital tomographic imaging with time-modulated pseudorandom coded aperture and Anger camera. J Nucl Med 16: 402–413

Kuhl D E, Abass S, Reivich M 1975 Computerized emission tomography and determination of local brain function. In: De Blanc H J, Sorenson J A (eds) Non-invasive brain imaging. Soc Nucl Med, New York, p 67

Kuhl D E, Edwards R Q 1963 Image separation radioisotope scanning. Radiology 80: 653–661

Kuhl D E, Edwards R Q 1964 Cylindrical and section radioisotope scanning of the liver and brain. Radiology 83: 926–936

Kuhl D E, Edwards R Q 1968 Reorganizing data from transverse section scans of the brain using digital processing. Radiology 91: 975–983

Kuhl D E, Edwards R Q 1970 The Mark III scanner: A compact device for multiple-view and section scanning of the brain. Radiology 96: 563–570

Kuhl D E, and Sanders T P 1971 Characterizing brain lesions with use of transverse section scanning. Radiology 98: 317–328

Kuhl D E, Hale J, Eaton W L 1966 Transmission scanning: a useful adjunct to conventional emission scanning for accurately keying isotope deposition to radiographic anatomy. Radiology 87: 278–284

Kuhl D E, Edwards R Q, Ricci A R et al 1973 Quantitative section scanning using orthogonal tangent correction. J Nucl Med 14: 196–200

Kuhl D E, Edwards R Q, Ricci A R, Yacob R J, Mich T J, Alavi A 1976 The Mark IV system for radionuclide computed tomography of the brain. Radiology 121: 405–413

Kuhl D E, Hoffman E J, Phelps M E et al 1968 Design and application of the Mark IV scanning system for radionuclide computed tomography of the brain. IAEASM–210/99

Kuhl D E, Phelps M E, Engel J P, Hoffman E J, Robinson G D Jr, MacDonald N S, Knowell

A P, Winter J 1978 Relationship of local cerebral glucose utilization and relative perfusion in stroke and epilepsy: Determination by emission computed tomography of ^{18}F-fluorodeoxyglucose and ^{13}N-ammonia. (Abstr) J Comput Assist Tomogr 2: 655

Kuhl D E, Pitts F W, Sanders T P, Mirshkin M M 1966 Transverse section and rectilinear brain scanning using ^{99m}-Tc pertechnetate. Radiology 86: 822–829

Kuhl D E, Reivich M, Alavi A et al 1975 Local cerebral blood volume determined by three-dimensional reconstruction of radionuclide scan data. Circulat Res 36: 610–619

Kwoh Y S, Reed I S, Truong T K 1977 Back projection speed improvement for 3-D reconstruction. IEEE Trans Nucl Sci 24, 5: 1999–2005

Ionn A, Cottrall M, and Simons H 1978 Experimental measurements of impulse response and noise for an emission computed tomography system. Eur J Nucl Med 4: 251–259

Lim C K, Chu D, Kaufman L 1975 Initial characterization of a multiwire proportional chamber positron camera. IEEE Nucl Sci NS 22: 388–394

Linuma T A, Nagai T 1967 Image restoration in radioisotope imaging systems. Phys Med Biol 12: 501–509

MacDonald B, Chang L T, Perez-Mendez V, Shiraishi L 1974 Gamma-ray imaging using a Fresnel zone plate aperture, multiwire proportional chamber detector, and computer reconstruction. IEEE Trans Nucl Sci NS-21

Mallard J R 1973 A radioisotope scanner for rectilinear, arc, transverse section and longitudinal section scanning. Br J Radiol 46: 262–271

Mallard J R et al 1977 Radionuclide transverse tomography of brain and trunk. XIV Int Congress of Radiology. Rio de Janeiro

Mandelkorn F, and Stark H 1978 Computerized tomosynthesis, serioscopy, and coded scan tomography. Appl Optics, 175–180

May R S, Akcasu Z, Knoll G E 1974 Gamma ray imaging with stochastic apertures. Appl Optics 13: 2589

Mersereau R M 1973 Recovering multidimensional signals from their projections. Comput Graph Image Process 2: 179–195

Miraldi F, Di Chiro G 1970 Tomographic techniques in radioisotope imaging with a proposal of a new device: the tomoscanner. Radiology 94: 513–520

Mirell S G, Anderson G W, Blahd W H 1976 A tomographic brain imaging system using compton-scattered gamma-rays. In: Medical radionuclide imaging. Proc Symp IAEA, Los Angeles, vol 1, pp 255–262

Muehllehner G, Wetzel R A 1971 Section imaging by computer calculation. J Nucl Med 12: 76–84

Muehllehner G, Atkins F, Harper P V 1977 Positron camera with longitudinal and transverse tomographic capabilities. In: Medical radionuclide imaging, IAEA, Vienna, vol 1, pp 291–307

Muehllehner G, Buchin N P, Dubek G H 1976 Performance parameters of the positron imaging camera. IEEE Nucl Sci NS 23: 528–537

Murphy P H, Thompson W L, Moore M L, Burdine J A 1979 Radionuclide computed tomography of the body using routine radiopharmaceuticals. 1—System characterization. J Nucl Med 20: 102–107

Myers M J, and Mallard J R 1964 Long focusing depth independent collimators for in-vivo radioisotope scanning. Int J Appl Radiat 15: 725–739

Myers M J, Keyes W I, Mallard J R 1973 An analysis of tomographic scanning systems. In: Medical radioisotope scintigraphy. IAEA, Vienna, vol 1, pp 331–345

Oliva L (ed) 1976 The new image in tomography. Proc of the Symposium Actualitatis Tomographiae, Genoa, Italy, Sept 11–13 1975 Excerpta Medica, Amsterdam

Oppenheim B E Jun 1974 More accurate algorithms for iterative three-dimensional reconstruction. IEEE Trans Nucl Sci NS-21(3): 72–77

Orthenberg H D, Devenney J, Kuhl D E 1976 Transverse section radionuclide scanning in cisternography. J Nucl Med 17: 924

Oying L 1976 Digital reconstruction of an object from its projections with applications in nuclear medicine. (Dutch with English summary) M Sc Thesis. Techn Univ Delft, Holland

Oying L 1977 Attenuation corrections for emission reconstructions and fan beam convolutions methods. Int Report Institute of Nuclear Med. Utrecht, the Netherlands

Paans A M J, Nickels R J, DeGraff E J, Vaalburg W, Reiffers S, Steenhoek A, Woldring M G 1978 A dual head Anger camera system for the imaging of positron-emitting radionuclides. Int J Nucl Med 5: 266–271

Pang S C, Genna S 1976 The effect of attenuation on reconstruction and statistical noise. J Nucl Med 17: 552

Pang S C, Genna S 1975 A Fourier convolution fan-geometry reconstruction algorithm: Simulation studies, noise propagation, and polochromatic degradation. In: Workshop on reconstruction tomography in diagnostic radiology and nuclear medicine, San Juan, Apr 17–19

Pang S C, Genna S 1979 The effect of Compton scattered photons on emission computerized tomography. IEEE, Trans Nucl Sci New Scientist 26: 2

Pang S C, Genna S 1979 Attenuation and induced spread function in ECAT. J Nucl Med 19: 745

Papoulis A 1965 Random variables, and stochastic processes, McGraw-Hill, New York, p 347

Patton J A, Brill A B, King P H 1973 Transverse section brain scanning with a multicrystal cylindrical imaging device. In: Freedman G S (ed) Tomographic imaging in nuclear medicine. Soc Nucl Med, New York, pp 28–42

Pelc N J, Chesler D A June 1979 Utilization of cross-plane rays for three-dimensional reconstruction by filtered back-projection. J Comput Assist Tomogr 3(3): 385–395

Phelps M E 1977 Emission computed tomography. Semin Nucl Med 7: 337–365

Phelps M E, Hoffman E J, and Kuhl D E 1976 Physiologic tomography. In: Medical radionuclide imaging. Proceedings of a Symposium in Los Angeles (IAEE), p 233

Phelps M E, Hoffman E J, Kuhl D E 1977 Physiologic tomography: A new approach to in vivo measure of metabolism and physiological function. In: Medical radionuclide imaging. IAEA, Vienna, vol 1, pp 233–253

Phelps M E, Hoffman E, Mullani M A, Ter Pogossian M M 1975 Transaxial emission reconstruction tomography coincidence detection of positron emitting radionuclides. In: DeBlanc H, Sorenson J (eds) Non-invasive brain imaging, computed tomography and radionuclides. Soc Nucl Med, New York, ch 7, p 87

Phelps M E, Hoffman E J, Mullani N 1976 Design and performance characteristics of a whole body transaxial tomograph. (PETT III). IEEE Nucl Sci 23: 516–522

Phelps M E, Hoffman E J, Gado M et al 1975 Computerized transaxial transmission reconstruction tomography. In: DeBlanc H, Sorenson J A (eds) Non-invasive brain imaging, computed tomography and radionuclides. Soc Nucl Med, New York, pp 111–146

Phelps M E, Hoffman E J, Hightill R et al 1977 A new emission computed tomograph for positron emitters. J Nucl Med 18: 603

Phelps M E, Hoffman E, Huang H et al 1975 Effect of positron range on spatial resolution. J Nucl Med 16: 649–652

Phelps M E, Hoffman E J, Huang S C et al 1978 ECAT: A new computerized tomographic imaging system for positron-emitting radiopharmaceuticals. J Nucl Med 19: 635–647

Phelps M E, Huang S C, Hoffman E J, Selin C S, Sideris K, Kuhl D E 1978 Validation of the noninvasive tomographic measure of regional cerebral glucose metabolism in man with ^{18}F-2-fluoro-2-deoxyglucose. (Abstr) J Comput Assist Tomogr 2: 656–657

Phelps M E, Hoffman E J, Mullani N A et al 1975 Application of annihilation coincidence detection to transaxial reconstruction tomography. J Nucl Med 16: 210–224

Phelps M E, Hoffman E J, Mullani N A, Higgins C S, Ter Pogossian M M 1976 Design considerations for a positron emission transaxial tomograph. (Pet III) IEEE Trans on Nucl Sc NS 23: 516

Phelps M E, Hoffman E J, Mullani N A, Higgins C S, Ter Pogossian M M 1977 Some performance and design characteristics of PETT III. In: Ter Pogossian et al (eds) Reconstruction tomography in diagnostic radiology and nuclear medicine. University Park Press, Baltimore, p 371

Phelps M E, Hoffman E J, Selin C, Huang S C, Robinson G D, MacDonald N, Schelbert H, Kuhl D E 1978 Investigation of ^{18}F-2-deoxyglucose for the measurement of myocardial glucose metabolism. J Nucl Med 19: 1311–1319

Preston K Jr, Onoe M 1976 Digital processing of biomedical images. Plenum Press, New York, pp 133–226

Radon J 1917 On the determination of functions from their integrals along certain manifolds. Berichte über die Verhandlungen der königlich Sächsischen Gesellschaft der Wissenschaften zu Leipzig. Mathematisch-Physische Klasse 69: 262–277 [Ger]

Ramachandran G N, Lakshminarayanan A V 1971 Three-dimensional reconstruction from radiographs and electron micrographs: applications of convolutions instead of Fourier transforms. Proc Natl Acad Sci USA 68: 2236–2240

Reed I S (Fellow IEEE), Kwoh Y S, Truong T K, Hall E L (Member IEEE) 1977 X-ray reconstruction by finite field transforms. IEEE Trans Nucl Sci 24 1: 893–899

Riederer S J, Pelc N J, Chesler D A 1978 The noise power spectrum in computed x-ray tomography. Phys Med Biol 23: 446–454

Robb R A, Greenleaf J F, Ritman E L et al 1974 Three-dimensional visualization of the intact thorax and contents: a technique for cross-sectional reconstruction from multiplanar x-ray views. Comput Biomed Res 7: 395–419

Robertson J S, Marr R B, Rosenblum B et al 1973 32 Crystal positron transverse section detector. In: Freedman G S (ed) Tomographic imaging in nuclear medicine. Soc Nucl Med, New York, pp 142–153

Rosenfeld D, Macovski A 1977 Time modulated apertures for tomography in nuclear medicine. IEEE Trans Nucl Sci NS-24, No 1

De Rosier D J, Klug A 1968 Reconstruction of 3-dimensional structures from electron micrographs. Nature (Lond) 217: 130–134

Rossmann K 1969 Point spread-function, line spread function, and modulation transfer function. Tools for the study of imaging systems. Radiology 93: 257–272

Rowe R W, Keyes W I 1976 Comparison of scanner and camera systems for quantitative single photon emission tomography. IEEE Trans Nucl Sc New Scientist 26, 2: 2768

Rowley P D 1969 Quantitative interpretation of three-dimensional weakly refractive phase objects using holographic interferometry. J Opt Soc Am 59: 1496–1498

Scudder H J 1978 Introduction to computer aided tomography. IEEE Procedures 66: 628–637

Shepp L A, Logan B F 1974 Some insights into the Fourier reconstruction of a head section. IEEE Nucl Sci NS 21: 21–43

Simons H A B, Lonn A H R, Cottrall M F 1976 Three dimensional image reconstruction from gamma-camera images. Proc 4th Int Conf Med Phys Ottawa, Canada, IOPM

Singleton R M, Ransom P L, Mittra R 1976 Digital imaging of Gamma-ray sources with depth information. IEEE Trans Biomed Eng BME–23, No 3

Smith P R, Peters T M, Bates R H T 1973 Image reconstruction from finite numbers of projections. J Phys A 6: 361–382

Synder D L, Cox J R 1977 Reconstruction tomography in diagnostic radiology and nuclear medicine. University Park Press, Baltimore

Sobel B E, Weiss E S, Welch M J et al 1977 Detection of remote myocardial infarction in patients with positron emission transaxial tomography and intravenous ^{11}C-palmitate. Circulation 55: 853–857

Soussaline F, Todd-Pokropek A E, Plummer D, Comar D, Loch C, Houle S, Kellershohn C 1979 The physical performance of a single slice positron tomographic system and preliminary results in a clinical environment. Eur J Nucl Med 4: 237–249

Steinback A, Macovski A 1976 Improved depth resolution in coded aperture gamma-ray imaging systems. IEEE Trans Nucl Sci NS–23, No 1

Sweeney D W, Vest C M 1973 Reconstruction of three-dimensional refractive index fields from multidirectional interferometric data. Appl Optics 12: 2649–2664

Syrota A, Comar D, Cerf M, Plummer D, Mazière, M, Kellershohn C 1979 ^{11}C-Methionine pancreatic scanning with positron emission computed tomography. J Nucl Med (in press)

Tanaka E, Iinuma T A 1975 Correction functions for optimizing the reconstructed image in transverse section scan. Phys Med Biol 20: 789–798

Tanaka E, Shimizu T, Iinuma T, Fukuhisa K 1973 Digital simulation of section image reconstruction. In: National Institute of Radiological Sciences, Annual Report 1972. Science and Technology Agency, Japan

Tank G et al 1978 Three dimensional reconstruction in planar positron cameras. IEEE Trans Nucl Sc N525: 196–201

Ter Pogossian M M 1977 Basic principles of computed axial tomography. Semin Nucl Med 7: 109–127

Ter Pogossian M M, Phelps M E, Brownell G L 1977 Reconstruction tomography in diagnostic radiology and nuclear medicine. University Park Press, Baltimore

Ter Pogossian M M, Phelps M E, Hoffman E J 1975 A positron emission transaxial tomograph for nuclear medicine imaging (PETT) Radiology 114: 89–98

Ter Pogossian M M, Mullani N A, Hood J et al 1978 A multislice positron emission computed tomograph (PETT IV) yielding transverse and longitudinal images. Radiology 128: 477–484

Ter Pogossian M M, Weiss E S, Coleman R E et al 1976 Computed tomography of the heart. Am J Roent 127: 79–90

Thompson C J, Meyer E, Yamamoto Y L 1978 Positron II: A high efficiency PET device for dynamic studies. J Comput Assist Tomogr 2: 650–651

Todd-Pokropek A E 1972 Two methods for improving section scanning. Strahlentherapie 72: 396–401

Todd-Pokropek A E 1972 The formation and display of section scans. In: Proceedings of Symposium of American Congress of Radiology, 1971, Excerpta Medica, Amsterdam, p 545

Todd-Pokropek A E 1973 Tomography and the reconstruction of images from their projections. In: Proc 3rd Int Conf data handling and image processing, Boston

Tothill P 1974 Limitations of the use of the geometric mean to obtain depth independence in scanning and whole body counting. Phys Med Biol 19: 382

Tretiak O J 1975 The point spread function for the convolution algorithm in image processing for 2D and 3D reconstruction from projection: Theory and practice in medicine and the physical sciences. Stanford Inst for Elect in Med and Op Soc of America, ThA5–1, Stanford, Calif

Tretiak O J, Ozonoff D, Klopping J et al 1971 Calculation of internal structure from multiple radiograms. In: Proc Two-Dimensional Digital Signal Processing Conference, Oct 6–8, 1971, Columbia Mo, IEEE NY, pp 6–2–1 to 6–2–3

Vainstein B K 1970 Finding the structure of objects from projections. Kristallografiya 15: 894–

902. Translated in Soviet-Physics—Crystallography, 1971 15: 781–787

Vallebona A 1931 Radiography with great enlargement (microradiography) and a technical method for radiographic dissociation of the shadow. Radiology 17: 340–341

Vasseur J P 1975 Relations between irradiation and image quality in reconstruction tomography. In: Workshop on reconstruction tomography in diagnostic radiology and nuclear medicine, San Juan, Apr 17–19

Walton P 1973 An aperture imaging system with instant decoding and tomographic capabilities. J Nucl Med 14: 861–863

Walters T E, Simon W, Chesler D A, Correia J A, Kiederer S T 1975 Radionuclide axial tomography with correction for internal absorption. Information processing in scintigraphy. Proc of the IVth Intern Conference Orsay, p 333

Weiss H, Klotz E, Linde R 1975 Deconvolution systems for coded aperture images at three-dimensional x-ray objects. Optics and Laser Tech 117–119

Woods J W, Ekstrom M P, Palmieri T M, and Twogood R E 1975 Best linear decoding of random mask images. IEEE Trans Nucl Sci NS–22

Wooley J L, Williams B, Verkatesh S 1977 Cranial isotopic section scanning. Clin Radiol 28: 517

Yamamoto Y, Thompson C J, Meyer E et al 1977 Dynamic positron emission tomography for study of cerebral hemodynamics in a cross section of the head using positron emitting 67-Ga EDTA and 77Kr. J Comput Assist Tomogr 1: 43–56

Yamamoto Y, Thompson C J, Meyer E et al 1977 Krypton-77 positron emission tomography for measurement of regional cerebral blood flow in a cross section of a head. Acta Neur Scand (Suppl) J6: 448

Zacher R 1975 Resolution limits for reconstruction tomography based on photon attenuation. In: Workshop on reconstruction tomography in diagnostic radiology and nuclear medicine, San Juan, Apr 17–19

Zatz L M 1975 The EMI scanner: Collimator design, polochromatic effects and selective material imaging. In: Workshop on reconstruction tomography in diagnostic radiology and nuclear medicine, San Juan, Apr 17–19

Ziedses des Plantes B G 1932 Eine neue Methode zur Differenzierung in der Röntgenographie (Planigraphie). Acta Radiol 13: 182–192

Zwick M, Zeitler E 1973 Image reconstruction from projections. Optik 38: 550–565

INDEX